Manual of
ENDOMETRIOSIS

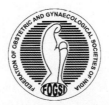

Federation of Obstetric and Gynaecological Societies of India

Manual of
ENDOMETRIOSIS

Kanthi Bansal
MD DGO FICOG

Director, Safal Fertility Foundation, Ahmedabad, Gujarat, India
Chairperson, Endometriosis Committee FOGSI
Clinical Secretary ISAR
Chairperson Accreditation Committee ISAR
Secretary Gujarat Chapter ISAR
Secretary ISAR 2014
Peer Reviewer JOGI
Peer Reviewer JRSCB
Special Invitee AOGS
Editor AOGS
E-mail: kanthibansal@gmail.com
Website: www.ivfbest.com

Foreword
Roy Homburg

A FOGSI Publication

JAYPEE BROTHERS MEDICAL PUBLISHERS (P) LTD
New Delhi • London • Philadelphia • Panama

Jaypee Brothers Medical Publishers (P) Ltd

Headquarters

Jaypee Brothers Medical Publishers (P) Ltd
4838/24, Ansari Road, Daryaganj
New Delhi 110 002, India
Phone: +91-11-43574357
Fax: +91-11-43574314
Email: jaypee@jaypeebrothers.com

Overseas Offices

J.P. Medical Ltd
83, Victoria Street, London
SW1H 0HW (UK)
Phone: +44-2031708910
Fax: +02-03-0086180
Email: info@jpmedpub.com

Jaypee-Highlights Medical Publishers Inc.
City of Knowledge, Bld. 237, Clayton
Panama City, Panama
Phone: +507-301-0496
Fax: +507-301-0499
Email: cservice@jphmedical.com

Jaypee Brothers Medical Publishers Ltd
The Bourse
111 South Independence Mall East
Suite 835, Philadelphia, PA 19106, USA
Phone: + 267-519-9789
Email: joe.rusko@jaypeebrothers.com

Jaypee Brothers Medical Publishers (P) Ltd
17/1-B Babar Road, Block-B, Shaymali
Mohammadpur, Dhaka-1207
Bangladesh
Mobile: +08801912003485
Email: jaypeedhaka@gmail.com

Jaypee Brothers Medical Publishers (P) Ltd
Shorakhute, Kathmandu
Nepal
Phone: +00977-9841528578
Email: jaypee.nepal@gmail.com

Website: www.jaypeebrothers.com
Website: www.jaypeedigital.com

© 2013, Federation of Obstetric and Gynaecological Societies of India

Inquiries for bulk sales may be solicited at: jaypee@jaypeebrothers.com

This book has been published in good faith that the contents provided by the contributors contained herein are original, and is intended for educational purposes only. While every effort is made to ensure accuracy of information, the publisher and the editor specifically disclaim any damage, liability, or loss incurred, directly or indirectly, from the use or application of any of the contents of this work. If not specifically stated, all figures and tables are courtesy of the editor. Where appropriate, the readers should consult with a specialist or contact the manufacturer of the drug or device.

Manual of Endometriosis

First Edition: **2013**

ISBN 978-93-5090-404-6

Printed at : Ajanta Offset & Packagings Ltd., New Delhi

Dedicated to

My son
Aditya

Contributors

Asha Baxi MS FRCOG FICOG (UK)
Director
Disha Fertility and Surgical Center
Indore, Madhya Pradesh, India

C Archana Devi MD
Consultant
Ramakrishna Nursing Home
Trichy, Tamil Nadu, India

Firuza Rajesh Parikh MD DGO DFP FCPS DIP NBE
Director, Department of Assisted Reproduction and Genetics
Jaslok Hospital and Research Center
Editor-in-Chief, Fertility and Sterility, Indian Edition
Mumbai, Maharashtra, India

Hrishikesh D Pai MD FCPS FICOG MSc (Clinical Embryology—USA)
Treasurer of FOGSI
Vice President of ISAR
President of Mumbai Obstetrics and Gynecological Society
Past Senior Vice President of FOGSI
Past President of Indian Society of Gynecological Endoscopists
Consultant IVF Expert
Fortis Bloom IVF Center, New Delhi/Mohali/Vashi and Lalavati Hospital
Mumbai, Maharashtra, India

Jaideep Malhotra MBBS MD
Consultant Infertility Specialist
Malhotra Nursing and Maternity Home
Agra, Uttar Pradesh, India

Kamini A Rao DGO DORCP DCH FRCOG (UK) MOBG (UK) FICOG
PGDNLE (UK) FANAMS
Director
Bangalore Assisted Conception Center (BACC)
Bengaluru, Karnataka, India

Kanthi Bansal MD DGO FICOG
Director, Safal Fertility Foundation, Ahmedabad, Gujarat, India
Chairperson, Endometriosis Committee FOGSI
Clinical Secretary ISAR
Chairperson Accreditation Committee ISAR
Secretary Gujarat Chapter ISAR
Secretary ISAR 2014
Peer Reviewer JOGI
Peer Reviewer JRSCB
Special Invitee AOGS Editor AOGS

Madhavi Panpalia MBBS MS (Obs & Gyne)
Clinical Associate
Department of Assisted Reproduction
Jaslok Hospital and Research Center
Mumbai, Maharashtra, India

Mandakini Parihar MD DGO FICOG
Vice President of FOGSI (2012)
Director, Mandakini IVF Center, Mumbai
Chairperson, Family Welfare Committee, FOGSI
Honorary Associate Professor
Department of Obstetrics and Gynecology
KJ Somaiya Medical College and Hospital
Mumbai, Maharashtra, India

Mekala D MD
Fellowship in GYN Medicine
Consultant Infertility Specialist in Reproductive Medicine
Bangalore Assisted Conception Center (BACC) Health Care Pvt Ltd
Bengaluru, Karnataka, India

Nandan Roongta DNB DGO DFP
Consultant Gynecologist
Bloom IVF Center
Lilavati Hospital
Mumbai, Maharashtra, India

Nandita Palshetkar MD FCPS FICOG
First Senior Vice President of FOGSI (2011)
Treasurer
Indian Association of Gynecological Endoscopists and
Mumbai Obstetrics and Gynecological Society
Member, Managing Committee of ISAR
Consultant IVF Expert
Fortis Bloom IVF Center, New Delhi/Mohali/Vashi and
Lilavati Hospital, Mumbai
Trustee, DY Patil Medical College
Mumbai, Maharashtra, India

Neeta Warty MD DGO Diploma in Endoscopy (Germany)
Gynecological Endoscopic Surgeon
Sanjeevni Endoscopic Center
Mumbai, Maharashtra, India

Nidhi Gupta MD
Associate Professor
Department of Obstetrics and Gynecology
SN Medical College
Agra, Uttar Pradesh, India

Parul J Kotdawala MD FICOG FICNCH
Diploma in Pelvicoscopy (Germany)
Honorary Endoscopic Surgeon and
Ex-Associate Professor
Department of Obstetrics and Gynecology
Vadilal Sarabhai Hospital
Ahmedabad, Gujarat, India

PM Gopinath MD DGO FMMC FICS FICOG MBA
Director
The Institute of Social Obstetrics
Government Kasturba Gandhi Hospital for
Women and Children
Chennai, Tamil Nadu, India

Prashant Joshi MD
Associate Professor
Department of Obstetrics and Gynecology
Adichunchanagiri Institute of Medical Sciences
BG Nagara, Karnataka, India

Pratap Kumar DGO MD FICOG FICS FICMCH
Professor
Department of Obstetrics and Gynecology
Kasturba Medical College
Manipal University
Manipal, Karnataka, India

Rajat Mohanty MD LLB
Senior Consultant
Department of Obstetrics and Gynecology
Shri Ramachandra Bhanj Medical College
Cuttack, Odisha, India

Ramesh B MD DGO DFP FCPS
Director
Dr Ramesh Hospital, Bengaluru
Consultant Gynecological Endoscopic Surgeon
Infertility and ART Specialist and
Urogynecologist
Bengaluru, Karnataka, India

Rishma Dhillon Pai MD DNB DGO FCPS FICOG
Consultant Gynecologist
Lilavati and Jaslok Hospitals, Mumbai
Board Member
World Endometriosis Society (WES)
Mumbai, Maharashtra, India

Rutvij Dalal MBBS MD DNB DGO
Fellow in Reproductive Medicine
Lilavati Hospital
Mumbai, Maharashtra, India

Sandip Datta Roy MS (Obs & Gyne)
Fellowship in Minimally Invasive Surgery (Gynecological Endoscopy)
Dr Ramesh Hospital and Research Center
Bengaluru, Karnataka, India

Shwetha Pramod MBBS DGO DNB (OBG) FIRM
Fellow in Infertility Medicine
Obstetrician and Gynecologist
Infertility Specialist
Radhakrishna Hospital
Bengaluru, Karnataka, India

Sonal Kotdawala MD
Kotdawala Women's Clinic
Ahmedabad, Gujarat, India

Sudipta Patnaik MD
Assistant Professor
Department of Physiology
Maharaja Krishna Chandra Gajapati Medical College
Berhampur, Odisha, India

Sujata Kar MD DNB
Kar Clinic and Hospital Pvt Ltd
Bhubaneswar, Odisha, India

T Ramani Devi MD DGO FICS FICOG
Consultant
Ramakrishna Nursing Home
Director
Janani Fertility Center
Trichy, Tamil Nadu, India

Vidya V Bhat MD DNB (Obs & Gyne) MNAMS FICOG
Obstetrician and Gynecologist
Sonologist and Laparoscopic Surgeon
Infertility Specialist
Radhakrishna Hospital
Bengaluru, Karnataka, India

Foreword

The very mention of the word endometriosis conjures up a series of questions. What is the etiology and pathophysiology? Why is the diagnosis so often missed or delayed? How should it best be treated? Do the milder forms of endometriosis cause infertility? What is the significance of adenomyosis?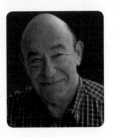

As with many enigmatic diseases, there is a plethora of hypotheses and therapeutic possibilities. In this *Manual of Endometriosis*, Dr Kanthi Bansal has gathered and presented the evidence which will undoubtedly provide an excellent guide to the practicing gynecologist.

The evolution of endometriosis is first explained leading to a description of the wide clinical spectrum. Does it really start from retrograde menstruation and, if so, why do some suffer from this and some not? All the problems of the diagnosis, and there are many, are then dealt with. Regarding the clinical spectrum and diagnosis, so much seems to depend on the location of the lesions. What should be done with ovarian endometrioma? When should they be surgically removed, punctured or left well alone? To what extent does endometriosis interfere with fertility? Is it only in the advanced stages? When should medical management be used and when is surgical management called for? These are various questions asked every day in practice. In this manual the contributors have rounded up the questions and answered them in a way which will provide an excellent guide.

Dr Kanthi Bansal is to be congratulated in having the courage and taking the bull by the horns by presenting and answering all the problems involved with this enigmatic disease. The readers of this manual will be the beneficiaries.

Roy Homburg
FRCOG
Professor of Reproductive Medicine
Maccabi Medical Services and Barzilai Medical Center, Israel
Head of Research
Homerton University Hospital
Queen Mary, London University
London, UK

Message

It gives me immense pleasure to write a few words for the *Manual of Endometriosis*. It must have been a simple and easy-to-understand format on such a difficult and complicated subject. I must congratulate Dr Kanthi Bansal for making such a great effort. All the chapters are carefully selected and written very methodically. There is clarity of thought and understanding of the subject which is evident in the writing of all the chapters.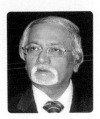

This book will immensely help the medical practitioners and members of FOGSI.

I wish Dr Kanthi Bansal, Chairperson of Endometriosis Committee, FOGSI and her team all the very best for their future endeavors. I will appreciate feedbacks and constructive critism from readers to present better reading material in future.

PK Shah
MD FICOG FCPS FICMU FICMCH DGO DSP
President
Federation of Obstetric and Gynaecological
Societies of India (FOGSI)

Message

This *Manual of Endometriosis*, dealing with the various aspects of the clinical, preventive and research aspects of the condition, I am sure, will highlight and answer a number of important questions related to the enigmatic condition that endometriosis has always been. I appreciate and applaud the efforts of the Endometriosis Committee of FOGSI and especially Dr Kanthi Bansal in bringing out this issue.

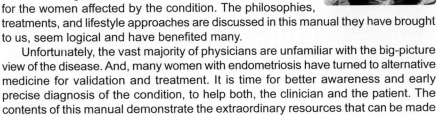

Dr Kanthi Bansal and the Endometriosis Committee are to be congratulated for their innovative advocacy work for the women affected by the condition. The philosophies, treatments, and lifestyle approaches are discussed in this manual they have brought to us, seem logical and have benefited many.

Unfortunately, the vast majority of physicians are unfamiliar with the big-picture view of the disease. And, many women with endometriosis have turned to alternative medicine for validation and treatment. It is time for better awareness and early precise diagnosis of the condition, to help both, the clinician and the patient. The contents of this manual demonstrate the extraordinary resources that can be made available to both.

Nandita Palshetkar
MD FCPS FICOG
First Senior Vice President of FOGSI (2011)
Treasurer
Indian Association of Gynecological Endoscopists and
Mumbai Obstetrics and Gynaecological Society
Member, Managing Committee of ISAR
Consultant IVF Expert
Fortis Bloom IVF Center, New Delhi/Mohali/Vashi and
Lilavati Hospital, Mumbai
Trustee, DY Patil Medical College
Mumbai, Maharashtra, India

Message

*Knowledge rests not upon truth alone, but upon error also —**Carl G Jung***

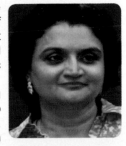

Endometriosis is an enigma and so many women suffer the pain of endometriosis and that affects the quality of life. All of us work individually for the betterment of women's health but joint effort is required by Government of India (GOI), medical associations, doctors and all the stakeholders for catalytic effect in improving reproductive health of our patients.

This book *Manual of Endometriosis* is essentially covering all the important topics from origins of endometriosis to the therapies. Modern management of endometriosis, endometriosis and infertility, surgery in endometriosis, pain management in endometriosis, surgical management of endometriosis, management of endometrioma, rectovaginal endometrioma, recurrent endometriosis and so many more well-covered topics make this book a must read.

This book on "endometriosis" is edited by Dr Kanthi Bansal, Chairperson of Endometriosis Committee of FOGSI has successfully managed to address all these issues related to endometriosis and I congratulate her on this excellent book and highlighting the importance of endometriosis.

Mandakini Parihar
MD DGO FICOG
Vice President of FOGSI (2012)
Director, Mandakini IVF Center, Mumbai
Chairperson, Family Welfare Committee, FOGSI
Honorary Associate Professor
Department of Obstetrics and Gynecology
KJ Somaiya Medical College and Hospital
Mumbai, Maharashtra, India

Message

It is a matter of great pride and privilege for Ahmedabad Obstetrics and Gynaeocological Society (AOGS) as an organization that one of its most respected member with illustrious academic career, Dr Kanthi Bansal has penned a *Manual of Endometriosis*. This disease is distressful condition for women suffering from it. The manual is such as, an epic book of endometriosis, where you find all the required answers for your queries related with the disease.

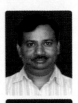

On behalf of AOGS, we wish her all the good luck for the warm acceptance by universe of academicians, including—private consultants, teachers, undergraduate and postgraduate students.

Dipesh Dholakia
MD
President
Ahmedabad Obstetrics and Gynaecological Society
Ahmedabad, Gujarat, India

Hemant Bhatt
MD LLB
Honorary Secretary
Ahmedabad Obstetrics and Gynaecological Society
Ahmedabad, Gujarat, India

Preface

The journey of life is mysterious, but the disease endometriosis is more mysterious than life itself! All aspects of endometriosis are still an enigma, right from incidence, diagnosis and management.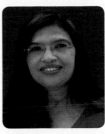

The Federation of Obstetric and Gynaecological Societies of India has taken a very important decision in giving this important field in gynecology, by forming a committee. I would like to thank the members, for electing me to be the first and founder Chairperson of this prestigious committee.

There are several activities organized by the endometriosis committee such as continuing medical educations (CMEs), workshops, international collaborations, adolescent health education for endometriosis, research and publications. Under the heading of publications, two important publications including the bulletin, Endometriosis Gen, a yearly publication and this book *Manual of Endometriosis* are published.

The book is drafted in a way to make it very interesting at the same time giving complete details in the topics to cover the subject in total. Almost all the topics related to endometriosis are covered from evolution, structure to function, diagnosis, endometrioma, infertility, adolescent endometriosis, recurrence, adenomyoma, scar endometriosis, rectovaginal endometriosis, coping with endometriosis to future thoughts.

I believe this book will be truly beneficial to postgraduate students, teachers and practicing doctors.

I feel this is a humble approach trying to unfold the mystery that is endometriosis.

Kanthi Bansal

Acknowledgments

My sincere thanks to all the contributors of this book for making it a dream come true for me. I am indebted to them for devoting their time in writing chapters for this manual despite their hectic schedule.

I thank Ms Khushboo Patel, for doing the coordinating work during the shaping up of this book.

Ms Aarti Vadinkar, deserves to be appreciated, for her input towards this book. I am glad that I have such an understanding family to back me. I thank my husband Dr Mukesh Bansal, my lovely children Suma and Aditya, for being so patient with me when I give their time to academic work.

The editorial staff of M/s Jaypee Brothers Medical Publishers (P) Ltd, New Delhi, India, have done a wonderful job, my heartfelt thanks to them.

Kanthi Bansal

Contents

Endometriosis: Evolution

◀ Asha Baxi, Manila Jain Kaushal

⮑ INTRODUCTION

Endometriosis is a chronic inflammatory disease, characterized by implantation and growth of endometrial tissue outside the uterine cavity. This disabling condition is considered one of the most frequent diseases in gynecology, affecting 15–20% of women in their reproductive life.

The first histological description of a lesion consistent with endometriosis was given by Carl Von Rokitansky, an Austrian pathologist in 1860.[1] By 1896, Cullen had suggested that endometriomas, or adenomyomas as he called these lesions, resembled the mucous membrane of the uterus.[2] Over the following 50 years adenomyoma and endometriosis were considered pathologies separate from the so-called 'hemorrhagic ovarian cysts', and it was not until 1921 that this condition was recognized to be of endometriotic origin. The year 2010 marked the sesquicentennial of the discovery and description of adenomyosis and endometriosis by Carl Rokitansky of Vienna.[3] The intervening 150 years have seen intense basic scientific and clinical research, and the diagnosis and treatment of millions of women worldwide. Yet there has been no scholarly history, and little mention of endometriosis and adenomyosis in historical compendiums of disease.

Sampson first described the disease formally in 1921.[4] Then he proposed the hypothesis that the origin of peritoneal endometrial implants was tissue delivered by the retrograde menstruation.[5] Retrograde menstruation is a nearly universal phenomenon among cycling women[5,6] but it is not clear why endometrial tissue will implant and grow in the peritoneal cavity of only a subgroup of women. These endometrial cells can respond to ovarian hormones and, therefore undergo cyclic menstrual changes with periodic bleedings. Several key steps are required to establish an endometriotic implant: presence of ectopic endometrial glands and stroma, attachment of endometrial cells to the peritoneum, invasion into the mesothelium, and survival and growth of the ectopic tissue.[7]

The history of endometriosis is reviewed in the light of today's clinical and pathological knowledge of this disease. Prior to Sampson's report in 1921, attention was focused on the enclosed type of endometriosis, sited deep in the pelvis and called adenomyosis externa. Sampson's first hypothesis, that rupture of an ovarian endometrioma caused superficial peritoneal endometriosis, was probably changed after this observation that the free, superficial peritoneal implants reacted like eutopic endometrium. These implants were recognized as implants from menstrual blood regurgitated into the pelvic cavity. Adenomyosis externa, ovarian endometrioma and peritoneal endometriosis then came to be regarded as the same disease. In the light of today's knowledge, it may be important to remember this progressive understanding in the nosology of what is now universally called pelvic endometriosis.

Evolution in Pathogenesis of Endometriosis

The pathogenesis of endometriosis is still subject to debate, although the condition has been known since 1860. Researchers have abundant theories about the causes of endometriosis, but have yet to prove any of them. These include retrograde menstruation/transplantation theory, coelomic metaplasia theory, anatomic abnormalities, genetic basis, environmental cause and altered cellular immunity. Among the theories concerning the pathogenesis of endometriosis three main concepts can be discerned **(Table 1.1)**.

The oldest concept is that endometriosis develops from the remnants of the Wolffian or Mullerian ducts, or alternatively, from metaplasia of the peritoneal or ovarian tissue.[8,9.]

In 1955, Levander and Normann introduced the induction theory.[7] This theory is based the assumption that specific substances which are released by the degenerating endometrium induce endometriosis from omnipotent blastoma, present in connective tissues. It is based on the assumption that endometriosis results from differentiation of mesenchymal cells, activated by substances released by degenerating endometrium that arrives in the abdominal cavity (the induction theory).[10,11]

A third concept is based on the transplantation and subsequent implantation of endometrial tissue.[5] This would imply transport of viable endometrial cells during menstruation through the Fallopian tubes into the abdominal cavity, implantation of these cells onto the peritoneum and the development of these cells into endometriosis (the transplantation or implantation theory). The implantation theory was originally neglected for a long time, because menstrual effluent was considered to contain only non-viable endometrial tissue and retrograde menstruation was thought to be a rare phenomenon.

Table 1.1: Pathogenesis of endometriosis—three main concepts

•	In situ development
•	Transplantation
•	Combination of in situ development and endometrial transplantation and implantation

The implantation theory explains the pathogenesis by deposition and subsequent growth of retrogradely shed viable endometrial cells. Transformation of mesothelium to endometrium-like tissue under the influence of products of regurgitated endometrium (induction) is a plausible alternative. In both models, cell adhesion molecules may play an important functional role.

Adequate animal models for endometriosis are not there. Rodents do not have spontaneous endometriosis which is not surprising since they do not have a menstrual cycle with a long luteal phase and menstruation. Also, primates are not an adequate model for endometriosis. The rhesus monkey only occasionally develops cystic ovarian endometriosis, possibly more after dioxin administration.[12] Also, in the baboon, there was failure to induce the more severe cystic or deep endometriosis.

It is likely that endometriosis is a common multifactorial disease, caused by an interaction between multiple gene loci and environment. Causes of immune or inflammatory deficiency may be related to the effects of stress on immune functioning, or may be genetically determined. The immune system, genetics and metaplasia are implicated in the pathogenesis of endometriosis. Women with endometriosis exhibit abnormally high humoral immune responsiveness and macrophage activation while showing diminished cell-mediated immunity with decreased T-cell and natural killer cell responsiveness. However, this may result from the presence of endometriosis rather than the cause.[13,14]

Chronic immunosuppression in combination with hormonal regulation may have facilitated the aberrant growth of endometrial tissue within the peritoneum. It seems that the genetical, environmental, immunological and hormonal factors interfere with each other and, implicating that a circle occurred could be responsible for the development and progression of endometriosis. However, the mechanism appears to require endometrium and retrograde menstruation in most cases of disease.

Pelvic endometriosis, the most common form of the disease, is associated with increased secretion of proinflammatory cytokines, neoangiogenesis, intrinsic anomalies of the refluxed endometrium and impaired function of cell-mediated natural immunity.[15] Recently, endometriosis has also been considered to be an autoimmune disease, owing to the presence of autoantibodies, the association with other autoimmune diseases and recurrent immune-mediated abortion. These findings are in apparent contradiction with the reduced cell-mediated natural immunity observed during the disease. Basic research on this field may lead to a better understanding of disease etiology. It is believed that some women's immune systems are unable to remove the fragments of endometrial tissue transported into the pelvic area, which can lead to endometriosis. Metaplasia, or changing from one normal type to another normal type of tissue to adapt to its environment, underlies another theory.[16] The endometrium and the peritoneum are derivatives of the same coelomic wall epithelium. Peritoneal mesothelium has been postulated to retain its embryologic ability to transform into reproductive tissue. Such transformation may occur spontaneously, or it may be facilitated by exposure to chronic irritation by retrograde menstrual fluid.

Evolution in Clinical Presentations and Diagnosis

Endometriosis is a late-comer in medical knowledge about diseases. Since endometriosis is an internal disease, it is not surprising that historically the symptoms were poorly understood. It was not until 1690 that an astute German physician, Daniel Schoen, published Disputatio Inauguralis Medica de Ulceribus Ulceri, in which he clearly described what we now know as endometriosis. In 1774, a Scottish physician wrote, "in its worst stages, this disease affects the well-being of the female patient totally and adversely, her whole spirit is broken, and yet she lives in fear of still more symptoms such as further pain, the loss of consciousness and convulsions." Indeed, that sounds like endometriosis!

Throughout the 18th century women were often considered to have "hysteria" rather than a gynecologic condition that caused pain. As for infertility, that was always blamed on the woman, but not specifically attributed to endometriosis. Recognition by the medical profession of endometriosis as a disease improved after it was clearly described by Dr Carl von Rokitansky in 1860. Since 1925, it has been known as "endometriosis," which combines "endometrium" (the lining of the uterus) with "-osis" (meaning abnormal). In this case, the endometrial tissue was found in an abnormal place.

In 1932, Hill reported the presence of aberrant endometrium at microscopy in a series of 135 patients who were operated-upon for some pelvic pathology. Amongst these cases, 20 had adenomyomas of the uterus and 115 had peritoneal endometriosis.[17] Pelvic pain related to menstruation was the principal reason for seeking relief through surgery and this usually happened some ten-years after the onset of disease.

Three different types of endometriosis were subsequently distinguished.

Peritoneal Endometriosis

In the 1980s, it became evident that peritoneal endometriosis has multiple appearances. These lesions may represent replacement of mesothelium by an endometrial epithelium or endometrial polyp formation.[18-20] The anatomic distribution of ectopic endometrium supported the hypothesis of retrograde menstruation as the primary model of development of endometriosis.[21] The clinical importance of even very small lesions was suggested when, in a prospective study of artificial insemination in women with minimal endometriosis, Jansen found reduced fecundability.[22] Awareness of the existence of subtle peritoneal endometriosis produced an increase in the diagnosis of endometriosis, although clinical significance of early lesions remained controversial.[23,24]

From all published evidence Evers, et al[25] concluded that peritoneal endometriosis appears to be a dynamic disease, especially in the early phase, when subtle, atypical lesions may emerge and vanish again. The final answer to the question whether and in which cases endometriosis is a progressive disease will have to come from long-term prospective investigations studying spontaneous evolution of peritoneal lesions without therapeutic interference.

Rectovaginal Endometriosis

As in the case of infertility, investigators found poor correlation between lesion characteristics or stage of disease and pelvic pain. A strong correlation between pelvic pain and the depth of invasion was described in the presence of implants more than 10 mm deep. In contrast with superficial peritoneal endometriosis, these lesions have a structure closely resembling the adenomyomas described by Cullen.[2] In the late 1990s, rectal endoscopic ultrasonography was proposed to diagnose the presence of deep bowel infiltration and select patients for surgery.[26]

Ovarian Endometriosis

Ovarian endometriosis can present itself as very early lesions, plaques with free-floating adhesions, deep non-cystic lesions and typical chocolate cysts with adhesions. In a detailed study of 29 ovary specimens with chocolate cysts, Hughesdon[23] found that in 90 percent of them the ovarian endometrioma was formed by a pseudocyst. The surface of the ovary is adherent, usually to the posterior side of the parametrium and part of the ovarian cortex is invaginated. Endometriotic tissue is found at the site of adhesion and a thin layer of superficial endometrium-like tissue extends to cover partially or fully the invaginated cortex. Hughesdon concluded that ectopic endometrium does not simply erode its way into the ovary: the ovary is actively invaginated, thus providing a pseudocyst mimicking a uterus.[27]

The prominent symptoms of the disease are chronic pelvic pain and infertility. However, some of the patients do not have clinical symptoms. Patients who have minimal disease would complain of severe pain, conversely patients who have severe lesions may not complain at all of pain.

The cause for the associated infertility and/or pain is poorly understood. Except for adhesions, the mechanisms of the associated infertility are not defined. Also for pain, there is lack of understanding that why so many of the typical, cystic, and deep lesions do not cause pain.

Evolution in Treatment

Medical Treatment

In 1953, Meigs[28] recommended early and frequent childbearing as prophylaxis of endometriosis. He wrote: "It is the author's belief that avoidance of endometriosis through early marriage and frequent childbearing is the most important method of prophylaxis". The availability, in the late forties, of a non-steroidal, synthetic estrogen, diethylstilbestrol (DES), prompted another line of experimental treatment for severe endometriosis. Karnaky[29] in 1945, reported apparently good results, achieving amenorrhea with increasing daily doses of up 100 mg/day of diethylstilbestrol (DES). In his series, five patients became pregnant after stilbestrol was discontinued. Two researchers Kistner[30] and Andrews[31] brought new concept of "pseudopregnancy", the artificial creation of a hormonal situation mimicking that occurring naturally during pregnancy" as a treatment for endometriosis. This was achieved by the first oral contraceptive ever marketed, Enovid (norethinodrel plus mestranol). Further new generation oral contraceptive pills were used. During the second part of the 20th century, a number of additional hormonal regimens have been proposed, the first being an antigonadotropic steroid, danazol.[32] Until the late 1980s, this agent was the standard medical treatment for endometriosis. The chief drawback with danazol is its androgenic properties. Interesting results have been obtained with the introduction of gestrinone, a steroid with androgenic, antiprogestinic and antioestrogenic activities. Given the results obtained with a mild antiprogestin like gestrinone, it was logical to expect even better results with the first "real antiprogestrogen", mifepristone. Ever since its introduction, Gonadotropin-releasing hormone agonists (GnRHa) have emerged as a primary medical therapy for patients with symptomatic disease, although secondary hypoestrogenic side effects may limit compliance. Add-back therapy is a means of surmounting this problem. Recent studies have demonstrated that the use of add-back enhances compliance and duration of therapy.[33] Leuprolide acetate, goserelin acetate and nafarelin acetate are all effective agents.

Oral contraceptives, androgenic agents, estrogens, progestins, antigonadotropic agents, antiprogestins and GnRHa have all been used successfully, although at the present time, the latter preparations are the most popular medical therapy for endometriosis. Recently levonorgestrel-releasing intrauterine system with a depot formulation of a GnRHa is used in the control of endometriosis-related chronic pelvic pain in patients with severe endometriosis.[34] Among the additional advantages of the LNG-IUS is the fact that it does not provoke hypoestrogenism and requires only one medical intervention (for its introduction) every 5 years. Thus, it is the treatment of choice for chronic pelvic pain associated endometriosis in women who do not wish to conceive.

Ovarian suppression by hormonal treatment appears not effective and should not be offered for infertile patients with endometriosis. This recommendation is based on a metaanalysis by Huges et al.[34] In addition, hormone suppression before or after surgical treatment of endometriosis is contraindicated since there is no evidence of increased effectiveness over that of surgery alone, and the treatment prolongs or delays the opportunity for conception to occur.

Surgical Treatment

Surgical treatment of severe endometriosis started in the early 1900's, when anesthesia had advanced enough that surgery was relatively safe. The surgical exploration and endoscopic access constitute major progress in the surgical management of endometriosis.

Technical improvements in laparoscopy quickly produced new information on endometriosis and expanded gynecological applications of endoscopic surgery, to the extent that in the early 1970s leading gynecologists in Europe and US concluded that laparoscopy is the preferred tool for diagnosis and surgery of endometriosis.[35]

During the last 35 years, gynecologic laparoscopy has evolved from a limited surgical procedure used only for diagnosis. Surgical therapy is appropriate, especially for advanced stages of the disease.

The laparoscopic approach offers a number of advantages over more conventional approaches. It causes precise destruction of lesions and adhesions, minimal bleeding and minimal damage to adjacent structures thus minimizing neoadhesions formation and nondrying of structures as occurs at laparotomy.

Open microsurgery therapy for endometriosis consists of a series of mini-operations performed under magnification using operating loupes. It emphasizes on limiting peritoneal damage and handling meticulous hemostasis and closure of raw areas without tension using finest non-absorbable suture.

Laparoscopy is an effective surgical approach with the goal of excising visible endometriosis in a hemostatic fashion. The goal of the surgery is to remove as much lesions as possible. The more aggressive approach to removal of implants and adhesions, increase the likehood of conception, particularly in patients with moderate and severe endometriosis with anatomical distortion.[36]

The treatment of infertility caused by endometriosis is surgical removal of endometriotic tissue or assisted reproductive technology. Peritoneal implants are resected or vaporized by means of an electric current or laser. Ovarian endometrioma and rectovaginal endometriotic nodules, however, can be removed effectively only with the use of full dissection. Surgical excision of the endometriomas carries a risk of reducing the oocyte pool of the patient which may add to her infertility problems. Ovarian reserve can be monitored by antimullerian hormone (AMH) levels in the serum in early follicular phase and could be of help to decide as of endometrioma should be removed before IVF or not. It is worthwhile to mention that surgery before IVF is suggested by ESHRE and the RCOG when ovarian endometrioma of > 4 cm in diameter is present[37] or there is suspicion of malignancy.

Endometriosis is often treated surgically upon diagnosis but with a higher rate of recurrence, suggesting that a combination of surgical and medical management might provide better outcomes. It is unfortunate that understanding of the disease has not progressed very far. This area may be of paramount importance in the near future in order to develop a therapy that could prevent or eradicate endometriosis rather than merely relieving the symptoms.

⮒ CONCLUSION

Endometriosis remains an enigma despite having been extensively studied. Although the exact etiology of endometriosis is unknown, several hypotheses about its origin exist. Multiple *in vitro* and *in vivo* models have been developed to study endometriosis. Over the last decade, great interest has been shown for the reconstruction of the path that led to the identification of endometriosis. Peritoneal endometriosis became the signature of endometriosis and the introduction of laparoscopy in the sixties provided a golden tool for the visual diagnosis and surgical therapy. While endometriosis remains an enigmatic disease, the introduction of new pharmacologic agents, such as GnRHa and newer endoscopic methods of surgical treatment, have facilitated and improved the overall management of this disease. Although now there are many medical and surgical treatments for endometriosis, the knowledge about the disease is still in its infancy. We know what it looks like, but we do not know why it is there. We know that in some women it is inherited, but we are just beginning to know what genes are involved.

⮒ REFERENCES

1. Von Rokitansky C. Ueber Uterusdrusen-Neubildung in Uterus- und Ovarial--Sarcomen. Ztschr KK Gesellsch der Aerzte zu Wien. 1860; 37:577-81.
2. Cullen TS. Adenomyoma uteri diffusum benignum. Johns Hopkins Hosp Bull. 1896; 6:133-7.
3. Benagiano G, Brosens I. Who identified endometriosis? Fertil Steril 2011;95:13-6.
4. Sampson JA. Perforating hemorrhagic (chocolate) cysts of the ovary. Arch Surg 1921;3:245-323.
5. Sampson JA. Peritoneal endometriosis due to the menstrual dissemination of endometrial tissue into the peritoneal cavity. Am J Obstet Gynecol. 1927;14:422-69.
6. Sampson JA. The development of the implantation theory for the origin of peritoneal endometriosis. Am J Obstet Gynecol. 1940;40:549-57.
7. Batt RE. Emergence of endometriosis in North America: a study in the history of ideas. Ph.D. dissertation. Buffalo (SA): University of Buffalo, State University of New York. 2008:109-13.
8. Ridley JH. The histogenesis of endometriosis. A review of facts and fancies. Obstet. Gynecol. Survey, 1968;23:1-23.
9. Lauchlan SC. The secondary Mullerian system. Obstet. Gynecoi. Survey, 1972;27: 133-46.
10. Levander G, Normann P. The pathogenesis of endometriosis. An experimental study. Acta Obstet. Gynecoi. Scand. 1955;34:366-98.
11. Merrill JA. Endometrial induction of endometriosis across Millipore filters. Am. J. Obstet. Gynecoi, 1966;94:780-90.
12. MacKenzie WF, Casey HW. Animal model of human disease. Endometriosis. Animal model: endometriosis in rhesus monkeys. Am J Pathol. 1975;80:341–4.

13. Gaetjii R, Lotzian S, Hermann G, et al. Invasiveness of the endometriotic cells *in vitro*. Lancet 1995;346:1463-4.
14. Dmowski WP, Braun D, Gebel. The immune system in endometriosis. In: Rock J., ed. Modern approaches to endometriosis. New York: Kluver Academic Publishers. 1991:97.
15. Badawy SZA, Cuenca V, Marshall L, et al. Cellular components in peritoneal fluid in infertile patients with and without endometriosis. FertiL.Steril., 1984;42:704-7.
16. Jones RK, Bulmer JN, Searle RF. Immunohistochemical characterization of proliferation, oestrogen receptor and progesterone receptor expression in endometriosis: a comparison of eutopic and ectopic endometrium in normal cycling endometrium. Hum. Reprod. 1995;10:3272-9.
17. Hill LL Jr. Aberrant endometrium. Am J Surg. 1932;18:303-21.
18. Vasquez G, Cornillie F, Brosens IA. Peritoneal endometriosis: scanning electron microscopy and histology of minimal pelvic endometriotic lesions. Fertil Steril 1984;42:696-703.
19. Murphy AA, Green WR, Bobbie D, dela Cruz ZC, Rock JA. Unsuspected endometriosis documented by scanning electron microscopy in visually normal peritoneum. Fertil Steril 1986;46:522-4.
20. Wiegerinck MA, Van Dop PA, Brosens IA. The staging of peritoneal endometriosis by the type of active lesion in addition to the revised American Fertility Society classification. Fertil Steril 1993;60:461-4.
21. Jenkins S, Olive L, Haney AF. Endometriosis: pathogenetic implications of the anatomic distribution. Obstet Gynecol 1986;67:335-8.
22. Jansen RP. Minimal endometriosis and reduced fecundability: prospective evidence from an artificial insemination by donor program. Fertil Steril 1986;46:141-3.
23. Jansen RPS, Russell P. Nonpigmented endometriosis: clinical, laparoscopic, and pathologic definition. Am J Obstet Gynecol. 1986;155:1154-9.
24. Stripling MC, Martin DC, Chatman DL, Vander Zwaag R, Poston WM. Subtle appearance of pelvic endometriosis. Fertil Steril 1988;49:427-31.
25. Evers JL, Land JA, Dunselman GA, van den Linden PJ, Hamiltion JC. 'The flemish giant', reflections on the defense against endometriosis, inspired by Professor Emeritus Ivo A. Brosens. Eur J Obstet Gynecol Reprod Biol 1998;81:253-8.
26. Hughesdon PE. The structure of endometrial cysts of the ovary. J Obstet Gynaecol Br Emp. 1957;64:481-7.
27. Meigs JV. Endometriosis; etiologic role of marriage age and parity; conservative treatment. Obstet Gynecol 1953;2:46-53.
28. Karnaky KJ. The use of' stilbestrol for endometriosis; preliminary report. Southern Med J 1948;41:1109-11.
29. Kistner RW. The use of newer progestins in the treatment of endometriosis. Am J Obstet Gynecol 1958;75:264-78.
30. Andrews MC, Andrews WC, Strauss AF. Effects of progestin-induced pseudopregnancy on endometriosis: clinical and microscopic studies. Am J Obstet Gynecol 1959;78:776-85.
31. Greenblatt RB, Dmowski WP, Mahesh VB, Scholer HF. Clinical studies with an antigonadotropin-Danazol. Fertil Steril 1971;22:102-12.
32. Surrey ES. Gonadotropin-releasing hormone agonist and add-back therapy: what do the data show? Curr Opin Obstet Gynecol. 2010;22:283-8.
33. Petta CA, Ferriani RA, Abrao MS, Hassan D, Rosa E, Silva JC, et al. Randomized clinical trial of a levonorgestrel-releasing intrauterine system and a depot GnRH analogue for the treatment of chronic pelvic pain in women with endometriosis. Hum Reprod 2005;20:1993-8.

34. Huges E, Brown J, Collins JJ, Farquhar C, Fedorkow DM, Vandekeckhove P. Ovulation suppression for endometriosis. Cochrane Database Syst Rev 2007;18;(3): CD000155.
35. Nezhat C, Crowgey SR, Garrison CP. Surgical treatment of endometriosis via laser laparoscopy. Fertil Steril 1986;45:778-83.
36. Cohen MR. Surgical laparoscopy in infertility. J Reprod Med 1975;15:51-3.
37. Verecellini P, Somigliana E, Vigano P, et al. Surgery for endometriosis associated infertility: a pragmatic approach. Human Reproduction 2009;24(2):254-69.

Endometriosis: Structure to Function

◖ Rajat Mohanty, Sudipta Patnaik

⊃ INTRODUCTION

Endometrium is a specialized form of mucous membrane lining the uterus. Endometrium contributes about 10% to the mass of the uterus. The uterus undergoes perhaps the most prominent ovarian steroid hormone dependent changes in structure and function of all the estrogen/progesterone target tissues.

Many of the cyclic changes in the uterine endometrium of the primate were described in the classic studies of Markee and his colleagues in the early 1940s. To document cyclic changes in endometrial morphology, Markee transplanted pieces of uterine endometrium into the anterior chamber of the eye in rhesus monkeys. The transplanted tissues became vascularized within 24 hours, and markee then made daily observations and drawings of the tissues under magnification, noting their size, composition, the location and size of vessels, etc. for up to as many as 72 consecutive cycles in one monkey. The transplanted tissue showed regular monthly changes in morphology, characterized by a growth cycle followed by a regression phase, with menstrual bleeding occurring towards the end of the regression period. Markee went on to examine the effects of a variety of hormones and drugs on the menstrual cycle.

⊃ PHYSIOLOGICAL ANATOMY

A basic knowledge of the fine structure of the endometrium, and of the relationship of the uterine blood supply to the endometrium is important to understand the function of the uterus and the uterine changes during nonfertile menstrual cycles.

The established functions of the endometrium is to limit the invasiveness of the implanting embryo so that it stays and is nourished in the endometrium and does not reach the myometrium. The glandular and vascular tissue of the endometrius support the physiological demand of growing fetus.

The endometrium is highly vascularized and has three components:
1. The luminal surface of the endometrium is covered by a simple cubodial/columnar epithelium. The epithelium is continous with mucous glands called uterine glands.

2. An underlying endometrial stroma is a very thick region of lamina propria (areolar connective tissue) which is densely cellular. These cells play important role during pregnancy and menstruation.
3. Endometrial (uterine) glands develop as invaginations of the luminal epithelium and extend almost to the myometrium.

The endometrium is divided into two layers, the stratum functionalis (functional layer), lines the uterine cavity and sloughs off during menstruation. The deeper layer the stratum basalis (basal layer), is permanent and gives rise to a new stratum functionalis after each menstruation.

Two kinds of arterial vessels pass through the myometrium to enter the endometrium. Branches of the internal iliac artery called uterine arteries supply blood to the uterus. Uterine arteries give off branches called arcuate arteries (shaped like a bow) that are arranged in a circular fashion in the myometrium. These arteries branches into radial arteries that penetrate deeply into the myometrium. Just before the branches enter the endometrium, they divide into two kinds of arterioles. Straight or basal arterioles which run for a short distance and supply the stratum basalis with the materials needed to regenerate the stratum functionales. Spiral arteries pursue a very tortuous course and end in subepithelial flexus of capillaries, which supply the stratum functionales and changes markedly during the menstrual cycle. Blood leaving the uterus is drained by the uterine veins into the internal iliac veins. The extensive blood supply of the uterus is essential to support regrowth of a new stratum functionales after menstruation, implantation of a fertilized ovum and development of the placenta **(Fig. 2.1)**.

About two-third of the luminal side of the endometrium (functional zone) is lost during menstruation. The basal one third of endometrium (stratum basal) remains after menstruation.

The Uterine Cycle

In human fetus, the uterine mucosa is capable of responding to steroid hormones by 20 weeks of gestation. Some of the uterine glands begin secreting material by the 22nd week of gestation. Endometrial development

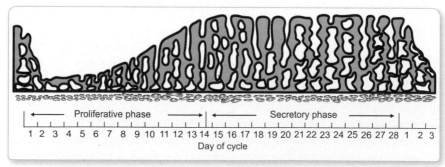

Figure 2.1: Changes in the endometrium during the menstrual cycle

in utero apparently occurs in response to estrogens derived from the maternal placenta. At 32 weeks gestation, glycogen deposition and stromal edema are present in the endometrium. An estrogen stimulation is withdrawn after delivery, the endometrium regresses, and at 4 weeks after birth, the glands are atrophic and lack vascularization. The endometrium remains in this state until puberty.

The Ovarian Hormones Drive the Morphological and Functional Changes of the Endometrium During the Monthly Cycle

The ovarian steroids—estrogen and progesterone—control the cycle monthly growth and breakdown of the endometrium. The three major phases in the endometrial cycle are: the menstrual, proliferative and secretary phases.

The menstrual phase: If the oocyte was not fertilized and pregnancy did not occur in the previous cycle, a sudden diminution in estrogen and progesterone secretion will signal the demise of the corpus luteum. As hormonal support of the endometrium is withdrawn, the vascular and glandular integrity of the endometrium degenerates, the tissue breaks down, and menstrual bleeding ensures, this moment is defined as day one of the menstrual cycle. After menstruation, all that remains on the inner surface of most of the uterus is a thin layer of non epithelial stromal cells and some remnant glands. However epithelial cells remain in the lower uterine segments as well as regions close to the fallopian tubes.

The proliferative phase: After menstruation, the endometrium is restored by about the fifth day of the cycle as a result of proliferation of the basal stromal cells on the denuded surface of the uterus (the zona basalis) as well as the proliferation of epithelial cells from other parts of the uterus. The stroma gives rise to the connective tissue components of the endometrium. Increased mitotic activity of the stromal and glandular epithelium continues throughout the follicular phase of the cycle and beyond, until 3 days after ovulation cellular hyperplasia and increased extracellular matrix result in thickening of the endometrium during the late proliferative phase. The thickness of the endometrium increases from 0.5 to as much as 5 mm during the proliferative phase.

Proliferation and differentiation of the endometrium are stimulated by estrogen that is secreted by the developing follicles. Estradial binds to a nuclear receptor on the endometrial cell and the activated receptor interacts with the hormone response elements of specific genes and modulates their transcription rates. Estrogen is believed to act on the endometrium in part through its effect on the expression of proto oncogenes that are involved in the expression of certain genes. Parts of the effect of estrogens is to induce the synthesis of growth factors such as the insulin like growth factors (IGFs) tumor growth factors (TGFs) and epidermal growth factor (EGF). These autocrine and paracrine mediators are necessary for maturation and growth of the endometrium. Estrogen causes the stromal components of the endometrium to become highly developed. Estrogen also induces the synthesis of progestin receptors in endometrial tissue.

Progesterone in contrast opposes the action of estrogen on the epithelial cells of the endometrium and functions as anti-estrogen. Progesterone inhibits epithelial cell proliferation, but promotes proliferation of the endometrial stroma.

The secretary phase: During the early luteal phase of the ovarian cycle the further antiestrogenic effect of the progesterone halts the proliferative phase of the endometrial cycle. Progesterone also stimulates the glandular components of the endometrium and thus induces secretory changes in the endometrium. The epithelial cells exhibit marked increase in secretory activity, indicated by increased amount of endoplasmic reticulum and mitochondria. These increases in synthetic activity occur in anticipation of the arrival and implantation of the blastocyst.

The early secretory phase of the menstrual cycle is characterized by the development of a network of interdigitating tubes within the nucleolus of the endometrial epithelial cells (nuclear channel system). Progesterone stimulates the development of this channel system, which provide a route of transport of mRNA to the cytoplasm.

During the middle to late secretory phase, there is still more increased secretory capacity of the endometrial glands. Vascularization of the endometrium increases, the glycogen content increases and the thickness of the endometrium increases to 5 to 6 mm. The endometrial glands become engorged with secretions. The glands appear tortuous and maximal secretory activity is achieved by approximately day 20 or 21 of the menstrual cycle **(Fig. 2.2)**.

The changes in the endometrium are not limited to the glands, they also occur in the stromal cells between the glands. Beginning 9 to 10 days after ovulation stromal cells that surround the spinal arteries of the uterus enlarge and develop eosinophilic cytoplasm with a prominent golgi complex and endoplasmic reticulum. This process is referred as predecidualization. The rounded decidual cells differentiate from spindle shaped fibroblast—like stromal cells under the influence of progesterone. As the stromal cells differentiate into decidual cells, their biochemical activity changes, and they form secretory products typical of decidual cells. Laminin, fibronection, heparin sulfate and type IV collagen surround matrices of these decidual cells. Multiple foci of these decidual cells spread throughout the upper layer of the endometrium and form a dense layer called the zona compacta. This spreading is so extensive that the glandular structures of the zona compacta become inconspicuous. Inflammatory cells accumulate around glands and blood vessels. Edema of the midzone of the endometrium distinguishes the compact area from the underlying zona spongiosa where the endometrial glands become more prominent.

3

Diagnostic Modalities of Endometriosis and their Pitfalls

◀ Nandita Palshetkar, Hrishikesh D Pai, Nandan Roongta

⊃ INTRODUCTION

Enigmatic is the word most used for describing the clinical entity of Endometriosis. Every clinician is intrigued by and wants to better define the condition in order to simplify matters for self and for the concerned patient. Is it or not to be labelled as endometriosis? This air of mystery around the condition and its associated diagnoses call for better defined diagnostic modalities, and awareness of their use.

This chapter attempts to highlight the contemporarily available diagnostic modalities, along with their advantages and pitfalls.

⊃ HISTORY

"The history of a science is the science itself"—Goethe

❖ The beginnings or the pathogenesis of the Mullerian diseases like endometriosis and adenomyosis, are all interrelated by virtue of their origin from the mesoderm that formed the anlage of the Mullerian ducts and the urogenital ridge.[1]

❖ During the late 18th and early 19th centuries, Europe experienced a philosophical and scientific reorientation necessary for the recognition of the chronic disease of endometriosis hidden within the female body.

❖ In the mid 19th century, Karl Freiherr von Rokitansky an antomical pathologist developed a research program that became the foundation of the 2nd Vienna Medical School, and wrote his magnum opus "Handbook of Pathological Anatomy." Rokitansky after his detailed and intellectual analysis of the macroscopic and microscopic anatomic features, discovered two new important diseases, adenomyosis and endometriosis.

❖ Then in the first half of the 20th century, a generation of European pathologists formulated various theories of pathogenesis, including von Recklinghausen's Wolffian theory. Across the Atlantic ocean, Thomas Cullen of the Johns Hopkins Hospital, challenged this Wolffian theory, and also closer to the origin of the theory, Robert Meyer, a former student disapproved his old master's Wolffian theory. DeWitt Casler presented the "Menstruating ovary" before the American Gynecological Society, inspiring John Sampson's theory of peritoneal implantation (1927) from perforating hemorrhagic cysts of the ovary. Iwanhoff-Meyers theory of coelomic metaplasia was also put forth.

❖ In the latter half of the 20th century, in around the early 1960s, the introduction of laparoscopy distinguished three different clinical presentations of endometriosis, peritoneal, deep adenomyotic and cystic ovarian.

❖ The 21st century saw endometriotic disease being recognised as a well-defined clinical entity, and today, it is known that viable endometrium reaches the peritoneal cavity during menses, activates the peritoneal immune system and elicits an inflammatory response. It is also known that occult microscopic endometrial implants are found submesothelially in visually normal peritoneum, even in women without identifiable endometriosis. The phase in between these two stages of development is still a mystery. Regurgitation and implantation of shed endometrium may not be the only origin of endometriosis, but also maybe invloved coelomic metaplasia. Epigenetic and environmental factors may also play a role.

⊃ PATHOLOGY

Endometriosis is defined as the presence of functional endometrial glands and stroma outside the uterine cavity.

Pathologically, though they may occur anywhere in the abdomen and pelvis, endometriotic lesions are usually confined to the pelvis with particular sites of predilection. Extra adnexal endometriotic deposits typically involve the broad ligaments, dome of the urinary bladder, distal ureters, rectouterine septum and pouch of Douglas. Serosal involvement of loops of small bowel within the pelvis and occasionally the serosal surfaces of the rectum is well-documented.

They range from microscopic foci to large hemorrhagic cysts and stellate pigmented patches. The most common type of involvement is endometriotic cysts within the ovaries, the result of repeated cyclical hemorrhage within deep deposits. Cyst characteristics typically include thick fibrous walled cysts with thick dark degenerate blood products, producing the characteristic chocolate cyst. They are often bilateral (50% of cases) and large (5–15 cm).[2]

The amount of pigment and the gross findings depend on:

❖ The duration of the disease: The amount of pigment increases with lesion age. Early lesions appear as white or yellow foci which gradually darken with repeated hemorrhage, leading to brown ecchymotic areas described as powder burns

❖ Pathological and clinical course

❖ The depth of tissue penetration by endometriotic deposits.

Repeated cycles of hemorrhage lead to fibrosis and subsequent adhesions between involved tissues potentially leading to distortion of the uterus, obliteration of the pouch of Douglas and small bowel adhesions.[3]

⊃ EPIDEMIOLOGY

Endometriosis is benign but complex, and its causes are probably multifactorial. Endometriosis is estimated to affect 1 in 10 women during the reproductive years, i.e. 6–10% of the general female population is affected by it. But amongst those women with pelvic pain or infertility, the prevalence rises to 35–50%.

Three main theories have been proposed:

A. Metastatic spread via retrograde menstruation, lymphatic and vascular spread and intraoperative implantation: Retrograde menstruation is well-documented at laparoscopy and up to 90% of women have bloody peritoneal fluid during menstruation.[4]

B. Metaplastic conversion of serosal surfaces into viable endometrial tissue.

C. Induction theory where shed retrograde endometrium induces endometrial differentiation of adjacent normal serosa[5] : Abnormalities of T-cell mediated cytotoxicity, B-cell function, natural killer cell activity and abnormal complement activation and growth factors almost certainly play a pivot role.[6]

⮥ CLINICAL FEATURES

Pelvic pain and infertility, the two most common clinically important sequelae of long standing endometriosis, are variably associated with endometriosis.

❖ Thirty to fifty percent of women with endometriosis are subfertile and 20% of infertile women have endometriosis.[7] The causal mechanism is thought to include impaired fallopian tube function due to adhesions and autoimmune factors[8]

❖ Pelvic pain is a common complaint with symptoms including dysmenorrhea, dyspareunia, chronic pelvic and low back pain and rectal discomfort.[8] If endometriotic deposits extend through the bladder or rectal wall, patients may present with hematuria, urinary frequency, tenesmus and rectal bleeding. Pain is not always cyclical as endometriotic deposits have a variable, often non cyclical response to circulating estrogen

❖ Involvement of the distal ureters may lead to distal ureteric fibrosis and obstruction with subsequent renal obstruction and flank pain

❖ Small bowel involvement may present with diarrhea and obstructive symptoms

❖ Involvement of the pleura results in pleuritic chest pain, pleural effusions, hemoptysis and pneumothorax

❖ Cyclical headaches from subarachnoid deposits and cutaneous bleeding from skin deposits have also been documented.[9,10]

⮥ DIAGNOSTIC EVALUATION

The only way to diagnose endometriosis is by laparoscopy or other types of surgery (Laparotomy, sigmoidoscopy, cystoscopy) with lesion biopsy. Hence, surgery is the gold standard in diagnosis since it permits direct visualization and tissue biopsies.

Clinical Evaluation

A detailed clinical history and examination can, in many patients, lead the physician to suspect endometriosis, and can be used as a screening test to identify patients requiring the "gold standard" diagnostic test of a laparoscopy. The common symptoms associated with endometriosis are dysmenorrhea, pelvic pain at other times of the menstrual cycle, and dyspareunia. But, these symptoms may occur in many different gynecological conditions. Also clinical evaluation of endometriosis is suboptimal due to the non specific physical findings. Localized tenderness, thickened or nodular uterosacral ligaments or rectovaginal masses and adnexal tenderness and masses may be found. The uterus is often retroverted from adhesions. The findings are however non-specific and may be absent in severe pelvic endometriosis **(Fig. 3.1)**.

Pitfalls of a Clinical Diagnosis

Relying solely on the symptoms and clinical assessment can lead to many unnecessary laparoscopies and the associated surgical risks. It is hence not recommended as an acceptable diagnostic or screening test.

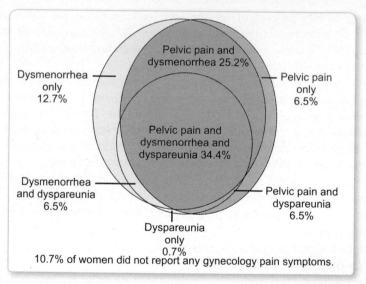

Figure 3.1: Prevalence and overlap of gynecologic pain symptoms that led to the surgical diagnosis of 940 women with endometriosis who participated in the OXEGENE study[11]

Diagnosis by Therapeutic Trial

Especially in adolescents with dysmenorrhea, where endometriosis is clinically suspected, medical treatment is appropriate before considering surgical evaluation and treatment. A trial of treatment with non-steroidal anti-inflammatory drugs (NSAIDs), ideally combined with an estrogen/progestin, or progestin only contraceptive is reasonable when the symptoms do not suggest an acute surgical condition.[12]

In adult women with chronic pelvic pain and suspected endometriosis also, some have advocated a medical therapy trail with gonadotrophin-releasing hormone (GnRH) agonist, when there is no other indication (e.g. an adnexal mass) for surgical treatment.

Pitfalls of a Therapeutic Trial—Retrospective Diagnosis

The pros and cons of a trial of therapy have to be weighed in adult women. The need for surgical intervention have to be thoroughly ruled out.

Surgical Evaluation

A. Endometrial Tissue Biomarkers

Recent research has highlighted endometrial biopsy (endometrial samples, endometrial fluid aspirates and menstrual effluent) as a potential diagnostic tool.[18,19,39]

Many aspects of endometrial function have been studied and found to differ endometriosis—angiogenesis, immune function, cytokines, proliferative potential of cell populations, and inflammatory factors.

❖ *Endometrial fluid analysis*: This represents a novel sample for proteomic analysis offering reliable, disease specific information on protein expression, facilitating the discovery of biomarkers for endometriosis

❖ *Secretory phase endometrium analysis*
  – Surface-enhanced laser desorption/ionization time-of-flight mass spectrometry analysis of secretory phase endometrium combined with bioinformatics puts forward a prospective panel of potential biomarkers with sensitivity of 100% and specificity of 100% for the diagnosis of minimal to mild endometriosis
  – The finding of small unmyelinated nerve fibers in the endometrium detected by staining with a rabbit polyclonal antibody to a protein gene product 9.5 (PGP 9.5).[18]

B. Laparoscopic Peritoneal Cavity Assessment

The earliest surgical method for diagnosing endometriosis was laparotomy.

With the advent of laparoscopy in the 1970s a relatively non-invasive method was available for diagnosing and treating a wide array of gynecological conditions, including endometriosis. Diagnostic laparoscopy with histologic examination of excised lesions is considered the 'gold standard' test for the diagnosis of endometriosis. The definitive diagnosis of endometriosis is based on the histological identification of endometrial glands and stroma. Also histologically associated factors like smooth muscle proliferation, fibromuscular hyperplasia, and inflammatory changes are indicative. Laparoscopy allows for concurrent treatment (Endometriotic cysts can be resected, deposits ablated and adhesions lysed **(Figs 3.2A to D)**, as well as diagnosis and local staging.

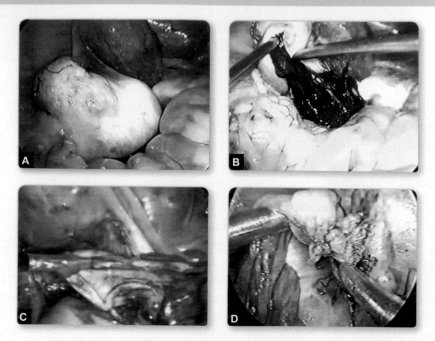

Figures 3.2A to D: Laparoscopic picture of ovarian endometrioma 'chocolate cyst' and adhesiolysis—(A) Diagnostic laparoscopy: left ovarian endometrioma, (B) Operative laparoscopy: left ovarian 'chocolate cyst' during excision, (C) Operative laparoscopy: cyst wall excision and (D) Operative laparoscopy: adhesiolysis

In recent years, transvaginal hydrolaparoscopy has been described as a possible alternative to diagnostic laparoscopy. It has been proposed as an office procedure with local anesthesia. A semirigid endoscope is used to visualize the Pouch of Douglas after entry via the posterior fornix using a Verres needle and instillation of warm saline. Disadvantages are that this technique does not allow for the visualization of the entire pelvis, and it is not possible to operate on any pathology found at the same time, through the used route. The rectum in particular is at-risk during entry. Also there is the risk of infection due to the vaginal route of entry. And it is risky in cases of rectovaginal endometriosis. It has hence not gained much popularity in clinical use.

At laparoscopy, disease extent is usually staged using the 1996 revised classification of Endometriosis[13] **(Table 3.1)**. A scoring is assigned to endometriotic lesions on the peritoneum and ovaries (based on size, location and depth), to posterior cul de sac endometriosis (partial and complete obliteration) and to adhesions on the ovaries and tubes (based on whether adhesions are filmy or dense, and the proportion of the tube or ovary covered).

Stage of the disease is divided into:
❖ Stage I (minimal): Score 1–5
❖ Stage II (mild): Score 6–15
❖ Stage III (moderate): Score 16–40
❖ Stage IV (severe): Score > 40

Table 3.1: American Society for Reproductive Medicine Revised Classification of Endometriosis

Peritoneum	Endometriosis	< 1 cm	1–3 cm	> 3 cm
	Superficial	1	2	4
	Deep	2	4	6
Ovary	R superficial	1	2	4
	Deep	4	16	20
	L superficial	1	2	4
	Deep	4	16	20
	Posterior cul de sac obliteration	Partial 4		Complete 40
	Adhesions	< 1/3 enclosure	1/3–2/3 enclosure	> 2/3 enclosure
Ovary	R filmy	1	2	4
	Dense	4	8	16
	L filmy	1	2	4
	Dense	4	8	16
Tube	R filmy	1	2	4
	Dense	41	81	16
	L filmy	1	2	4
	Dense	41	81	16

If the fimbriated end of the fallopian tube is completely enclosed, change the point assignment to 16
(*Courtesy:* Reproduced from Revised ASRM classification. Fertil Steri. 1997;67:819)

The pathology of the endometriotic lesion can vary widely. The appearances change depending upon the stage of their life cycle. Early lesions are red lesions, comprising early active endometriosis, with much associated inflammation. The mature black lesions are the classic chocolate cysts, composed of concentration of blood pigments from successive bleeds in response to cycling hormonal levels overtime. The final stage of the proposed life cycle of the endometriotic lesion is the white lesion, old burnt out endometriosis which has largely been replaced by collagen and scar tissue. There have been discussions regarding invisible microscopic endometriosis, lesions that are so small that they cannot be identified even under direct magnified vision with the laparoscope. A range of techniques have been described, including thermocoagulation test (endometriosis containing peritoneum turns brown rather than white after thermocoagulation, due to the hemosiderin content), methylene blue painting, and laparoscopic spectral analysis with blue light, in order to detect and remove these otherwise invisible endometriosis areas.

The classification systems at present do not make distinctions between these different types of lesions.

Another clinical tool, the Endometriosis fertility index (EFI)[14] that grades the condition from 0–10 (with 0 representing the poorest and 10 the best prognosis) was proposed in 2009. The key element of the new staging system, is a numerical measure of functional anatomy, based on careful assessment of the tubes (extent of serosal injury, mobility and patency), fimbriae (extent of injury, architecture) and ovaries (size, extent of surface injury). The EFI score attempts to predict the pregnancy rates in patients—with surgically documented endometriosis—who attempt non-IVF conception.

The classification most commonly used in clinical practice is descriptive and relatively simple:[12]

❖ Minimal Endometriosis: Isolated superficial disease on the peritoneal surface with no significant adhesions
❖ Mild Endometriosis: Scattered superficial disease on the peritoneal surface and ovaries, totalling less than 5 cm in aggregate, with no significant adhesions
❖ Moderate endometriosis: Multifocal disease, both superficial and invasive, that may be associated with adhesions involving the fallopian tubes and/ or the ovaries
❖ Severe endometriosis: Multifocal disease, both superficial and invasive, including large ovarian endometriomas, usually associated with adhesions, both filmy and dense, involving the fallopian tubes, ovaries, and cul de sac.

Pitfalls of a surgical diagnosis
❖ Despite being the gold standard of diagnosis in the condition, laparoscopy is a minimally invasive procedure requiring general anesthesia.
❖ The accuracy of the surgical diagnosis appears to rely heavily on both the experience and surgical skills as also the quality of the laparoscopic equipment.
❖ Laparoscopy is associated with a 1 in 10,000 mortality risk. The risks are magnified even further by women with established endometriosis, who often require several laparoscopies over the course of their reproductive life due to the high rate of recurrence despite surgical treatment. It also involves potential complications (such as damage to the bowel, bladder, and hemorrhage if large blood vessels are damaged) as well as procedural costs, and hence non-invasive screening methods are used for clinical purposes.[15]

Non-invasive screening methods: There is often a delay of an average 7–12 years, in making the diagnosis, mainly due to the non-specific nature of the associated symptoms and the need to verify the disease surgically.

C. Peripheral Biomarkers[16,31]

A biomarker that is simple to measure could help clinicians to diagnose (or at least exclude) endometriosis; it might also allow the effects of treatment to be monitored. If effective, such a marker or panel of markers could prevent unnecessary diagnostic procedures and/or recognize treatment failure at an early stage.

Current evidence suggests that endometriosis likely induces local and systemic inflammatory processes. Numerous studies have focused on markers of inflammation in an effort to find less invasive methods for diagnosing endometriosis. Detection of such a marker may result in an earlier diagnosis of endometriosis than can be made by the rather non-specific symptoms, and may replace the invasive surgical procedures to verify the disease. A biomarker could also be used to identify early signs of therapeutic efficacy or disease recurrence, as symptomatic relief or aggravation usually is hard to quantify. However, as the benefits of treating women with asymptomatic endometriosis are unclear, it is likely that any biomarker would be used only to investigate women with symptoms suggestive of endometriosis. Therefore, a prospective biomarker needs to distinguish women with endometriosis from women with similar presentations (for example, dysmenorrhea, pelvic pain or subfertility).

The commonly used biomarkers today are CA-125, Interleukin-6 and the neutrophil—lymphocyte ratio.

The following is a list of biomarkers being studied for their potential use for endometriosis screening **(Fig. 3.3)**.

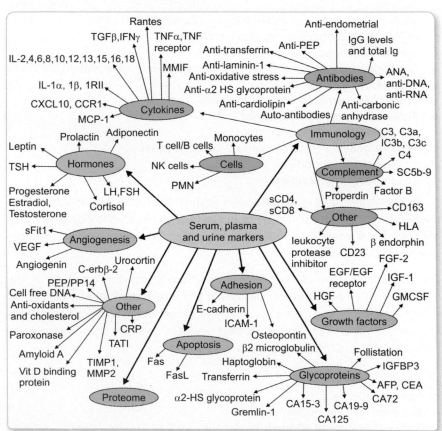

Figure 3.3: Spider diagram depicting putative biomarkers[16] (*Courtesy*: May K, et al. Hum Reprod. Update 2010;16:651-74)

Cytokines: Raised levels have been observed in endometriosis especially at an advanced stage.

The most studied cytokines have been interleukin-6 (IL-6) and tumor necrosis factor-alpha (TNFα).

❖ Interleukin-6
❖ Interleukin-8
❖ Tumor necrosis factor-alpha (TNFα)
❖ Monocyte chemotactic protein-1 (MCP-1)
❖ Interferon gamma
❖ Other cytokines: IL-1α / IL-1 receptor antagonist / IL-1 soluble receptor type II / IL-1β / TGFβ / macrophage migration inhibitory factor (MIF)
❖ Intracellular cytokines.

Antibodies: A great deal of interest has focused on circulating antibodies that may be a marker of endometriosis or involved in disease pathogenesis, especially because the interaction of the immune system with the endometrium is thought to have a major influence on how, and if, the disease develops.

❖ Total immunoglobulin
❖ Antiendometrial antibodies: The diagnostic accuracy of endometrial antibody testing appeared favorable with a sensitivity of 83% and specificity of 79%. Autoantibodies may also be affected by treatment
❖ Specific antibodies
❖ Antibodies against progestogen-associated endometrial protein (PEP) and endometrial glycoproteins
❖ Antibodies against carbonic anhydrase
❖ Antibodies to collagen, albumin and IgG
❖ Antibodies against transferrin
❖ Autoantibodies against markers of oxidative stress
❖ Antilaminin-1 antibodies
❖ Anticardiolipin antibodies.

In summary, some autoantibodies appear promising candidates as biomarkers for endometriosis. However, further work is required to elucidate which antigens are triggers for some of these autoantibodies, to refine laboratory testing for the disease.

Cell populations: One of the mechanisms that is probably involved in the development of endometriotic lesions is the interaction between sloughed endometrial tissue and the immune system. Consequently, various populations of immune cells have been studied to gain insights into the disease pathogenesis, and test their utility as biomarkers.

❖ T cells
❖ B cells
❖ Natural killer cells
❖ Macrophages/monocytes
❖ Polymorphonuclear neutrophils[17]
❖ Neutrophil-lymphocyte ratio.

Other immunology:
❖ C3c and C4
❖ SC5b-9—the membrane attack complex
❖ Mononuclear cell β-endorphin levels
❖ Soluble CD4
❖ CD23, an IgE receptor that also exists in a soluble form
❖ Soluble HLA class I and II were significantly lower in women with endometriosis.

Glycoproteins: The majority of studies have looked at glycoproteins which have been assessed in the past as 'tumor markers' because of their association with malignant disease.
❖ Cancer antigen 125: CA-125 is a high molecular weight glycoprotein. Although best known as a marker for epithelial ovarian cancer, its use is extensively studied over the last 20 years, as an endometriosis marker too. Elevated CA-125 levels have been observed in serum, menstrual effluent, and the peritoneal fluid (PF) of women with endometriosis. CA-125 may also be helpful in the detection of unusual presentations of endometriosis: for example, measuring CA-125 levels in women presenting with recurrent pneumothorax may identify thoracic endometriosis.

Pitfalls of a CA-125 as a marker for endometriosis:
– Although CA-125 is often elevated in advanced endometriosis, it may be more accurate at diagnosing women with later stages of disease only. Levels tend to be higher in women with endometriomas.
– The low sensitivity and specificity of this assay limits its usefulness for detecting minimal and mild disease.
– Also, it has not shown a correlation with disease response to treatment. Nor it has been found useful in the follow-up of patients with advanced endometriosis and initially elevated CA-125 levels.
– Due to its wide distribution particularly in the female pelvis, serum levels are elevated in a variety of benign and malignant disorders, particularly gynecological conditions. For example, endometriosis, uterine fibroids, adenomyosis, and pelvic inflammatory disease.
– The type of assay used to detect CA-125 may also affect its clinical performance.
❖ CA19-9
❖ CA15-3
❖ CA-72 (also known as TAG72)
❖ Other glycoproteins
– Serum transferrin
– α2-HS glycoprotein
– Alpha-fetoprotein (AFP)
– Carcinoembryonic antigen (CEA)
– Beta-2 microglobulin
– Haptoglobin-β (Hpβ) chain isoforms

- Follistatin
- Gremlin-1.

Cell adhesion:
* Intracellular adhesion molecule-1 (ICAM-1)
* Other
  - Soluble E-cadherin levels
  - Osteopontin, a glycoprotein involved in interactions between integrins, known to be expressed in the endometrium.
  - Soluble VCAM-1
  - P-selectin and E-selectin levels

Growth factors:
* Insulin-like growth factor-I (IGF-I)
* IGFBP3 is a protein that regulates the transport of IGF and influences the growth of endometrial cells
* Granulocyte macrophage colony-stimulating factor (GM-CSF), a growth factor that stimulates stem cells to produce granulocytes and monocytes.

Proteomics: In the area of biomarker discovery, proteomic techniques are proving particularly powerful tools to identify protein 'fingerprints' in blood or tissues that may be markers of disease. In the study of endometriosis, it would be the study of the gene expression profile of the endometriotic endometrium and the eutopic endometrium. From patterns of expression, individual peptides or proteins that are present or absent (or up-or down-regulated) in various disease states can be identified and assessed as possible biomarkers. Alternatively, the actual protein/peptide pattern itself can be used as a distinctive marker of disease presence.

The search for a differential serum protein expression in endometriosis attempts to identify specific peptide and protein patterns to diagnose endometriosis, mainly using two-dimensional electrophoresis (the classical method), and mass spectrometry [mainly matrix-assisted lazer desorption and ionization time-of-flight (MALDI) and surface-enhanced laser desorption/ionization time-of-flight mass spectrometry (SELDI-TOF MS)].

Proteomic technologies are providing innovative ways to identify bio-markers of disease and together with genetic profiling, they may be of use in identifying diseases by their protein fingerprints. However, the time and cost associated with these technologies currently prohibit their widespread use.

Hormones:
* Prolactin
  An association between galactorrhea and endometriosis was first identified over 30 years ago, which led to further investigation of the role of prolactin (PRL) in endometriosis. Timing of sampling is particularly important for prolactin, as levels have a diurnal pattern. One study showed that the 8 am

decline in prolactin levels (seen in healthy women) failed to occur in women with endometriosis.

- ❖ Pituitary hormones
  - – LH levels
  - – TSH
  - – Follicle stimulating hormone
- ❖ Steroids
  - – Progesterone
  - – Estradiol
  - – Testosterone
  - – Cortisol
- ❖ Leptin.
- ❖ Adiponectin was found to be significantly lower in women with endometriosis.

Angiogenesis: Several studies have sought to identify a link between endometriosis and pro-angiogenic factors in serum or urine—principally vascular endothelial growth factor (VEGF)—which may have use as biomarkers.

- ❖ VEGF levels
- ❖ Serum angiogenin (a polypeptide that stimulates angiogenesis) have been identified in women with endometriosis; however, this difference was only seen during the follicular phase of the cycle
- ❖ Raised urinary soluble Flt-1 levels (a VEGF receptor) have been noted in endometriosis patients, although there was no overall difference in serum levels. Interestingly, significantly higher urine and serum sFlt-1 levels were identified in women with earlier stage disease.
- ❖ Fibroblast growth factor-2 (FGF-2)
- ❖ Soluble epidermal growth factor (EGF) receptor
- ❖ Platelet-derived growth factor (PDGF)
- ❖ Serum Hepatocyte growth factor (HGF), a protein with important roles as a mitogen and chemoattractant for endothelial cells: levels were initially found to be elevated in women with endometriosis. Levels did not change throughout the cycle, but did correlate with disease stage (levels in Stages I–II were lower than in Stages III–IV disease).

Apoptosis: Soluble fas ligand (sFasL) levels in serum: Cells expressing fas undergo apoptosis on interaction with other cells expressing fas ligand. However, it also exists in a soluble form, due to cleavage from the cell surface by matrix metalloproteinases.

Other:
- ❖ C-reactive protein (CRP), an acute phase protein used widely to monitor inflammatory and infectious processes.
- ❖ Urocortin is a peptide belonging to the corticotrophin releasing hormone family, known to be expressed in the endometrium.

❖ Antioxidant and cholesterol levels:
  – Serum paroxonase-1 (PON-1)
  – High-density lipoprotein
  – Total cholesterol, triglycerides, low-density lipoprotein and lipid peroxidises.
❖ Circulating free DNA
❖ Vitamin D binding protein
❖ Phosphoenolpyruvate (PEP)
❖ Endometrial protein PP14 (related to PEP)
❖ Tumor-associated trypsin inhibitor (TATI) is a polypeptide known to be associated with gynecological neoplasms.
❖ Proto oncogene c-erbB-2
❖ Serum amyloid A (an acute phase protein)
❖ Serum tissue inhibitor of metalloproteinase-1 (TIMP-1) levels
❖ Serum matrix metalloproteinase-2 (MMP-2).

Genetic markers: Research is also being conducted on potential genetic markers associated with endometriosis so that a saliva-based diagnostic may replace surgical procedures for basic diagnosis. However, this research remains very preliminary.

Discussion

Establishing a correct diagnosis of endometriosis is often problematic, because the presenting symptoms can be non-specific and associated with a number of different conditions. Imaging methods such as transvaginal ultrasound and magnetic resonance imaging may help to identify ovarian endometriomas or a rectovaginal endometriotic nodule, but they have no value in diagnosing peritoneal endometriosis. Consequently, it is recommended that pelvic endometriosis should be diagnosed surgically.

An accurate blood or urine test could avoid the need for an invasive procedure, or at the very least could enable symptomatic women to be screened. It has previously been suggested that a biomarker may be of most clinical use in specific subgroups of women with endometriosis. For example, women with symptoms consistent with Stages I–II disease may benefit from laparoscopic treatment if endometriosis is present. However, for those women with the same symptoms but no endometriosis, the risks of laparoscopy may outweigh the benefits. As such, this may be the group of women in whom a biomarker test might be most useful.

Another role for a biomarker would be to identify early signs of therapeutic efficacy, other than symptom relief itself, which is so difficult to measure. Such a molecule would be vitally important for novel drug design and early clinical studies. In addition, as recurrence rates of up to 50% after 5 years have been reported, it would be desirable if a biomarker or a panel of biomarkers could predict the likelihood of disease recurrence. This could lead to different therapeutic approaches depending on the outcome of the test.

Till date, there have been identified over 100 possible biomarkers that have been investigated; however, none of these have been clearly shown to be of clinical use. Some have undoubtedly shown promise as diagnostic tools, but further research needs to be conducted to establish their true value in clinical practice.

It is worth noting that surgery often plays a vital role in the treatment of endometriosis. Furthermore, it may also be of importance in the management of other conditions which present in a similar manner (e.g. tubal infertility). The use of a biomarker may well be tempered in these circumstances, but it may still help to reduce the need for diagnostic surgery in some women, enable monitoring of the disease progression by non-surgical methods, and potentially allow for better preoperative assessment of women with endometriosis.

Finally, the majority of the studies included in our review focused on assessing the diagnostic performance of single biomarkers. Realistically, however, a reliable diagnostic tool for endometriosis is likely to consist of a panel of biomarkers, not a single molecule. Ultimately, with more studies investigating the use of technologies such as genomics, proteomics and metabolomics, it can be expected that a panel of molecules or a typical profile of gene or protein expression will in the future help to distinguish between patients with and without disease. In combination with imaging techniques, such a panel of biomarkers may indicate which women need a laparoscopy and eliminate countless unnecessary operations. Future, larger well-designed studies together with increased knowledge of the pathogenesis of endometriosis are essential to improve overall health-related quality of life for patients suffering from this debilitating disease.

In conclusion, peripheral biomarkers show promise as diagnostic aids, but further research is necessary before they can be recommended in routine clinical care. Panels[32, 33, 40] of markers including both substance concentrations and genetic predisposition may allow increased sensitivity and specificity of any diagnostic test.

D. Radiological Evaluation

The clinical presentation of endometriosis is variable and patients may be referred for imaging of a number of systems.[29, 34]

The role of radiology is mainly two fold. In the case of adnexal cysts, radiological characterization has an important role in confirming the etiology as endometriotic and excluding other, particularly neoplastic causes of adnexal masses. As with all imaging, radiological appearances are correlated with clinical information including serum enzymes. This is particularly important as both endometriosis and ovarian neoplasia can cause raised serum CA-125 levels. The second role of radiology is to identify and locally stage disease presence and extent as well as to identify and quantify complications such as adhesions and tubal pathology.

1. **Plain film radiography, intravenous urography and radiographic bowel imaging.**
   - In thoracic endometriosis, pleural lesions are invariably right sided and lead to cyclical hemothorax and pneumothorax. The rarer lung parenchymal lesions have no sided predilection and may result in cyclical hemoptysis. Chest X-ray findings include pneumothorax, ill defined lung nodules and pleural effusions, and are non specific for endometriosis.[21]
   - Intravenous urography (IVU) may identify involvement of the distal ureters with subsequent fibrosis and stricture, leading to a degree of ureteric obstruction. Full thickness endometriotic bladder implants may be seen as filling defects within the opacified bladder during late stages of the IVU exam.
   - Serosal deposits on pelvic small bowel (estimated to occur in 12–37% of patients with endometriosis)[20] may lead to fibrosis and adhesions between bowel loops, identified on small bowel follow through. Serosal involvement of the sigmoid colon and upper rectum may be seen as areas of extra mural stricturing and tethering on double contrast barium enema studies.

2. **Contrast enhanced computed tomography (CECT)**
   The role of CT scanning in endometriosis is limited to problem solving. While CT scanning is useful in diagnosing lung endometriomas and endometriomas in surgical scars in the abdominal wall, these are rare, and the exception rather than the rule. Patients with other complications may present with bowel obstruction from adhesions and strictures, hydronephrosis from ureteric obstruction and also pelvic pain from ruptured endometriomas.

   Pitfalls of CT diagnosis:
   - CECT identifies these complications of endometriosis, but is generally non specific regarding the underlying cause.
   - In the diagnosis of the more common ovarian endometriomas, the CT scan has little utility due to its poor ability to discriminate differences in soft tissue.
   - As for peritoneal endometriosis, it has no use at all at present due to the relatively poor tissue differentiation of pelvic organs and related structures.
   - The associated ionizing radiation dose is also a factor particularly as most patients are relatively young.

3. **Ultrasonography**
   The lack of ionizing radiation and relatively easy access makes ultrasonography the first imaging modality utilized in the investigation of endometriosis.[22,23] The only widely accepted use of ultrasound in diagnosing endometriosis is in the detection of ovarian endometriomas.

Endometriomas or 'chocolate cyst' may be unilateral or bilateral, and maybe associated with reduced mobility of the ovary. Bilateral endometriomas may be seen stuck together behind the uterus as kissing ovaries. They may be uni- or multilocular with thin or thick septations present. The contents of old blood, give a typical ground glass apprearance with low-level echoes, though rarely they may be anechoic, mimicking functional ovarian cysts.

Comparing with other adnexal lesions, endometriomas are more commonly bilateral and multiple. Further, an adnexal cyst that resolves on follow-up examination is likely to have been an acute hemorrhagic or functional cyst.

Transabdominal scanning (TAS) allows the detection of abdominal free fluid, identification of dilated small bowel loops in small bowel obstruction and allows the total extent of endometriomas to be assessed as these are often large and may be incompletely imaged on transvaginal scans.

Transrectal ultrasound combined with the instillation of vaginal saline, helps in the diagnosis of deep infiltrating rectovaginal endometriosis.

Transvaginal scanning (TVS) with a high frequency endoluminal probe allows detailed assessment of the pelvis. The most important role in endometriosis is the characterization of adnexal cysts and masses. TVS can thus help in identifying women with advanced endometriosis, and can detect ovarian endometriomas, but cannot image pelvic adhesions or superficial peritoneal foci of disease. TVS has 90% or higher sensitivity and almost 100% specificity for the detection of endometriomas.

2D ultrasound with additional information provided by the 3D and 4D technology along with Doppler assessment of the blood flows, can help in the delineation of adenomyosis and adnexal masses, along with assisting in the differential diagnosis of the same (**Figs 3.4A to D**).

Attention is particularly given to:

❖ *Internal echogenicity*: The highest single predictor for endometriosis is the presence of small mural echogenic foci present in 35% of endometriomas and only 6% of non endometriomas.[24] They most likely represent cholesterol deposits within the cyst wall from repeated hemorrhage. There is a wide overlap in appearances between endometriomas and acute hemorrhagic cysts, dermoids and cystic neoplasms. Acute hemorrhagic cysts typically evolve into more complex cysts due to clot retraction and fibrin stranding and generally resolve within six to eight weeks. Dermoids typically demonstrate calcification, fat fluid levels and multiple hyperechoic areas from materials such as hair and sebum. If the cyst demonstrates internal soft tissue components, a neoplasm must be ruled out.

❖ *Wall morphology*: Cyst wall thickness has no diagnostic value as 20% have nodular wall thickening, typically associated with ovarian neoplasia.[23]

❖ Effects on surrounding tissues [22]

❖ Elicitation of site-specific tenderness with the ultrasound probe.

Transvaginal or transrectal ultrasonography can be especially helpful when deeply infiltrating disease involving the bladder, the uterosacral ligaments, or the rectovaginal septum is suspected.

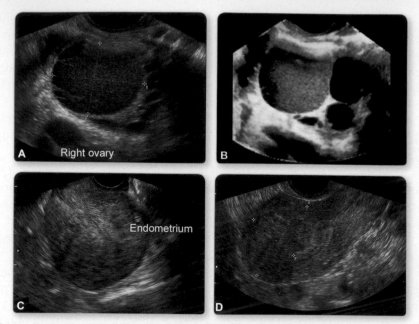

Figures 3.4A to D: Ultrasound images in endometriosis— (A) 2D TVS: Ovarian endometrioma, (B) 3D rendering of the ovarian endometrioma, (C) 2D TVS: An intense speckling of the endometrium—adenomyosis, and (D) 2D TVS: Focal adenomyosis

Pitfalls of ultrasound diagnosis:

❖ USG remains a poor test for endometriosis on the whole, apart from the detection of endometriomas and large deep infiltrative deposits.

❖ Due to their complex appearance and wide overlap with other adnexal lesions, endometriotic lesions are considered the most difficult to diagnose confidently on sonography alone and short-term USG follow-up or MRI is often utilized in conjunction with clinical assessment and serum enzyme markers.

❖ These types of imaging require considerable expertise and technology, not available in most centers.

❖ There are subjective elements involved (e.g. pain elicitation).

4. Magnetic resonance imaging

MRI scanning may have a role in tertiary centers in planning surgery for suspected deep infiltrating disease diagnosed at laparoscopy, and is increasingly used to determine the location and depth of endometric lesions prior to considering surgery. This helps in appropriate counselling of the patient regarding specific risks of the required surgery (e.g. bowel involvement, involvement of the ureters in deep infiltrating disease). Also a skilled team of surgeons could be organized for the anticipated surgery (e.g. laparoscopic colorectal surgeon, urologist, laparoscopic trained gynecologist).

MRI pelvis for endometriosis is best performed after day 8 of the cycle. A peristaltic inhibitor should be administered intramuscularly, and both T1 and T2-weighted images should be taken, with and without fat-suppression in T1 weighted images, and before and after administration of gadolinium contrast. The use of contrast enhanced imaging is usually reserved for cases of suspected adnexal malignancy, otherwise gadolinium contrast offers no additional diagnostic value.

Adnexal endometriotic cysts-endometriomas (Figs 3.5A to C):
Ovarian endometriomas are primarily diagnosed by ultrasound which is the imaging modality of choice, but MRI is being promoted as the second line investigation if the features on ovarian mass on ultrasound are difficult to interpret. MRI is used in both the characterization of endometriotic cysts and in the identification of extra adnexal aspects of endometriosis. MRI can detect endometriomas due to the characteristic hyperintensity in both T1 and T2 weighted images (due to old blood in 'chocolate cyst') and use of fat-suppressed T1 images to diffentiate it from a cystic teratoma. Sensitivity of 90% and specificity of 98% have been reported for MRI diagnosis of endometriomas. But these values can be highly operator dependent. The main advantage over TVS is that MRI can distinguish more reliably between acute hemorrhage and degenerated blood products. But like TVS, though MRI can help in the detection and differentiation of ovarian endometriomas from other cystic ovarian masses, it cannot reliably image small peritoneal lesions.

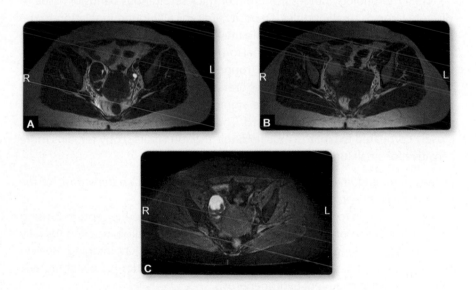

Figures 3.5A to C: Sequence of MRI images in a case of ovarian endometriomas: (A) Transaxial T1 weighted MRI image showing endometriomas, (B) Transaxial T2 weighted MRI image showing endometriomas, and (C) Transaxial T1 weighted fat saturated image showing endometriomas

Extra adnexal endometriosis-endometriotic implants, fibrosis and complications:
Extra adnexal endometriotic deposits appear as areas of nodular or plaque like areas of fibrosis which are of low signal intensity on both T1 and T2 weighted imaging. Fat suppression narrows the dynamic signal range and accentuates differences in tissue signal. Fat suppression is important in the evaluation of endometriosis. It suppresses the signal from normal pelvic tissues, improving the sensitivity of MRI in the detection of small lesions and improves its specificity as fat containing lesions such as dermoids demonstrate significant signal loss and can be eliminated from the differential diagnosis.[25] For the detection of peritoneal implants, MRI is superior to TVS, but still identifies only 30–40% of the lesions observed at surgery. For the detection of disease documented by histopathology, MRI is approximately 70% sensitive and 75% specific.

MRI plays an important role in the identification of extra adnexal endometriosis and subsequent complications.[26] Deposits have variable signal characteristics. They may appear similar to normal endometrium which is typically high signal on T2 and low signal intensity on T1 weighted images. With repeated cycles of hemorrhage and fibrosis, lesions demonstrate low signal intensity on both T1 and T2 weighted sequences. Occasionally, they appear as high signal lesions on all pulse sequences. Non-fibrotic implants may enhance following contrast administration but this is neither sensitive nor specific and as already mentioned, postcontrast images are not routinely obtained.[27]

Their morphology ranges from thin or thick serpiginous bands of tissue to discrete large or small nodules. Deposits are typically found in relation to the peritoneal reflections of the broad ligaments, rectovaginal septum and pouch of Douglas. Involvement of the vaginal fornices is well-documented. Thickening of the uterosacral ligaments and round ligaments is often seen. Serosal deposits on small bowel loops, distal ureters, dome of the urinary bladder and pelvic large bowel, particularly the sigmoid colon can be identified. Rectal involvement is increasingly detected. The identification of these deposits is closely correlated to laparoscopic findings, though laparoscopy remains more sensitive for small (under 2 mm) sized deposits.

Rectovaginal endometriotic nodules and deep infiltrating endometriosis of the uterosacral ligaments.
It is often possible to identify deposits within the rectouterine septum causing sharp retroversion of the uterus. Adhesional small bowel obstruction (usually incomplete and long standing) can be identified on LFOV imaging. Review of the distal ureters is important as it allows identification of distal ureteric stricturing and subsequent hydronephrosis.

Occasionally, deposits in relation to the sacral plexus may be identified as a cause of chronic intractable pelvic and lower limb pain.[28] Cutaneous deposits in relation to the umbilicus, previous laparoscopy ports, laparotomy scars and episiotomy incisions can be identified. Within the pelvis, particularly at the level of the pelvic floor, areas of peritoneal fibrosis lead to loculated fluid collections, unlike non endometriotic collections which tend to be free.

This application of MRI is seeing great enthusiasm of use in patients with symptoms suggestive of deep infiltrating lesions, owing to the poor ability of USG to detect endometriosis in these locations, combined with relative difficulty in detection of subperitoneal lesions even with laparoscopy.

Scarring and obstruction to the fimbrial ends of the uterine tubes
This could lead to hydrosalpinx and is an important radiological finding as it is a potentially treatable significant factor in associated subfertility.

Adenomyosis[30]
Adenomyosis can be better differentiated from fibroid uterus on MRI **(Figs 3.6 and 3.7)**. Adenomyotic lesions images sometimes mimic malignancies such as leiomyosarcoma and endometrial stromal sarcoma. High-resolution MR imaging at 3T demonstrates anatomically detailed structures and may improve diagnostic accuracy in differentiating adenomyosis from such mimics. Cine MR imaging is useful in differentiating transient myometrial contraction from focal adenomyosis.

Pitfalls of MRI diagnosis:
❖ High cost and low availability: Since symptoms are not a good screening method for the actual presence of endometriosis, it would mean that if MRI was employed for every symptomatic patient, it would be a very costly exercise.
❖ Need for considerable expertise in the interpretation of the MRI scans of the female reproductive tract.

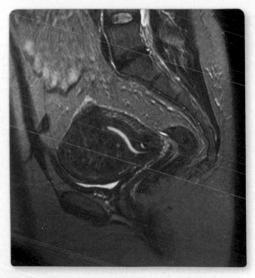

Figure 3.6: MRI image: Classical focal adenomyosis (anteriorly)

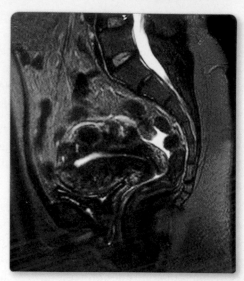

Figure 3.7: T2 weighted MRI image: Posterior well-defined rounded fibroid with anterior adenomyosis showing a markedly thickened junctional zone.

5. Other imaging modalities

❖ Immunoscintigraphy employing radiolabelled OC-125 antibody binding to areas of CA-125 expression. The specificity is low at 33% due to widespread expression of CA-125 by benign gynecological pathology.

❖ Positron emission tomography(PET): Increased uptake on PET scanning may be due to associated inflammation than presence of endometriosis per se.

❖ These methods hence have no clinical role in diagnosing endometriosis at present.

⊃ CONCLUSION

Careful clinical evaluation can identify women likely to have endometriosis but cannot establish the diagnosis. Serum biomarkers like CA-125 levels may provide corroborative evidence of the disease, but the sensitivity of the test is too low to make it an effective screening tool. Increasingly, transvaginal ultrasonography and MRI are used as adjuncts to laparoscopy with histologic examination, which remains the gold standard for the investigation and surgical management of patients with endometriosis. TVS and MRI are both highly sensitive and specific for the detection of ovarian endometriomas, but cannot reliably image peritoneal implants of the disease. In patients with a suspected adnexal mass, imaging is used to both confirm this and to characterize the lesion, enabling confirmation of its endometriotic nature in many cases and exclusion of malignancy in others. Whilst the identification of extra adnexal endometriosis by sonography remains anecdotal, MRI is becoming an increasingly important tool in the localization of deposits within the pelvis, allowing more accurate preoperative staging and providing a road map of disease to the surgeon. Advances in MRI imaging such as SFOV dedicated high resolution imaging of the rectum and the introduction of the multidisciplinary approach in many endometriosis centers promise exciting advances in the diagnosis and management of this often long-term debilitating condition.

⊃ REFERENCES

1. Ronald E Batt. A history of endometriosis. New York. Springer 2011.
2. Woodward P, Sohaey R, Mezzetti P. Endometriosis: radiologic-pathologic correlation. From the archives of the AFIP; Radiographics. 2001;21:193-216.
3. Crum CP. The female genital tract. In: Cortran RS, Kumar V, Collins T, eds. Robbins pathologic basis of disease. 6th ed. Philadelphia, Pa: Saunders 1999:1057-9.
4. Olive DL, Schwartz LB. Endometriosis. N Engl J Med. 1993;328:1759-69.
5. Liu DTY, Hitchcock A. Endometriosis: its association with retrograde menstruation, dysmenorrhoea and tubal pathology. Br J Obstet Gynaecol. 1986;93:859-62.
6. Badawy SZA, Cuenca V, Stitzel A, Jacobs RDB, Tomar RH. Autoimmune phenomenon in infertile patients with endometriosis. Obstet gynaecol. 1984;63:271-5.
7. Eskanazi B, Warner M. Epidemiology of endometriosis. Obstet Gynaecol Clin North Am. 1997;24:235-58.
8. Schenken RS. Endometriosis. In: Scott JR, Di Sala PJ, Hammond CB, Spellacy WN,eds. Danforth's obstetrics and gynaecology. 8th ed. Philadelphia, Pa: Lippincott Williams and Wilkins 1999:669-76.
9. Thibodeau LL, Prioleau GR, Manuelidis EE, Merino MJ, Haefner MD. Cerebral endometriosis: case report. J Neurosurg. 1987;66:609-10.
10. Hawayek LH, Abdulla FR. Cutaneous abdominal nodule after caesarean delivery. American Family Physician. 2009;80(12):1483.
11. Ninet Sinaii, Katherine Plumb, Louise Cotton, et al. Differences in characteristics among 1,000 women with endometriosis based on extent of disease. Fertility and Sterility. 2008;89(3):538-45.
12. Marc A Fritz, Leon Speroff. Clinical Gynecologic Endocrinology and Infertility. Philadelphia. Lippincott Williams & Wilkins, 2010.
13. American Society for Reproductive Medicine. Revised American Society for Reproductive Medicine classification of endometriosis: Fertility and Sterility. 1997;67(5):817-21.
14. G David Adamson, David J Pasta. Endometriosis fertility index: the new, validated endometriosis staging system. Fertility and Sterility. 2010;94(5):1609-15.
15. Juan Gracia-Velasco, Botros RMB Rizk, Botros RMB Rizk. Endometriosis current management and future trends. Jaypee Brothers Publishers, 2010.
16. May KE, Conduit-Hulbert, Villar J, Kirtley V, Kennedy SH, Becker CM. Peripheral biomarkers of endometriosis: a systematic review. Hum Reprod Update. 2010; 16(6): 651–74.
17. SiHyun Cho, Hanbyoul Cho, Anna Nam, Hye Yeon Kim, et al. Neutrophil-to-lymphocyte ratio as an adjunct to CA-125 for the diagnosis of endometriosis. Fertility and Sterility. 2008;90(6):2073-9.
18. Al-Jefout M, Dezarnaulds G, Cooper M, Tokushige N, Luscombe GM, Markham R, Fraser IS. Diagnosis of endometriosis by detection of nerve fibres in an endometrial biopsy: a double blind study. Hum Reprod. 2009;24(12):3019-24.
19. Bokor A, Debrock S, Drijkoningen M, Goossens W, Fülöp V, D'Hooghe T. Quantity and quality of retrograde menstruation: a case control study. Reprod Biol Endocrinol. 2009;30(7):123.
20. Clement PB. Diseases of the peritoneum. In: Kurman RJ, (ed). Blaustein's pathology of the female genital tract. 4th edition. New York: Springer-Verlag, 1994:660-80.

21. Joseph J, Sahn SA. Thoracic endometriosis syndrome: new observations from an analysis of 110 cases. Am J Med. 1996;100:164-70.
22. Guerriero S, Ajossa S, Paoletti AM, Mais V, Angiolucci M, Melis GB. Tumor markers and transvaginal ultrasonography in the diagnosis of endometrioma. Obstet Gynecol. 1996;88:403-7.
23. Volpi E, De Grandis T, Zuccaro G, La Vista A, Sismondi P. Role of transvaginal sonography in the detection of endometriomata. J Clin Ultrasound. 1995;23:163-7.
24. Patel MD, Feldstein VA, Chen DC, et al. Endometriomas: diagnostic performance of US. Radiology. 1999;210:739-45.
25. Dmowski WP, Lesniewicz R, Rana N, Pepping P, Noursalehi M. Changing trends in the diagnosis of endometriosis: a comparative study of women with pelvic endometriosis presenting with chronic pelvic pain or infertility. Fertil Steril. 1997;67:238-43.
26. Togashi K, Nishimura K, Kimura I, Tsuda Y, Yamashita K, Shibata T, et al. Endometrial cysts: diagnosis with MR imaging. Radiology. 1991;180:73-8.
27. Ascher SM, Agrawal R, Bis KG, Brown ED, Maximovich A, Markham SM, et al. Endometriosis: appearance and detection with conventional and contrast-enhanced fat suppressed spin echo techniques. J Magn Reson Imaging. 1995;5:251-7.
28. Chamie LP, Blasbalg R, Goncalves MO, Carvalho FM, Abrao MS, de Oliviera IS. Accuracy of magnetic resonance imaging for diagnosis and preoperative assessment of deeply infiltrating endometriosis. Int J Gynaecol Obstet. 2009;106(3):198-201.
29. Grasso RF, Di Giacomo V, Sedati P, et al. Diagnosis of deep infiltrating endometriosis: accuracy of magnetic resonance imaging and transvaginal 3D ultrasonography. Abdom Imaging. 2010;35(6):716-25.
30. Takeuchi M, Matsuzaki K. Adenomyosis: usual and unusual imaging manifestations, pitfalls, and problem-solving MR imaging techniques. Radiographics. 2011;31(1):99-115.
31. Mabrouk M, Elmakky A, Caramelli E, Farina A, Mignemi G, Venturoli S, Villa G, Guerrini M, Manuzzi L, Montanari G, De Sanctis P, Valvassori L, Zucchini C, Seracchioli R. Performance of peripheral (serum and molecular) blood markers for diagnosis of endometriosis. Arch Gynecol Obstet. 2011.
32. Agic A, Djalali S, Wolfler MM, Halis G, Diedrich K, Hornung D. Combination of CCR1 mRNA, MCP1, and CA125 measurements in peripheral blood as a diagnostic test for endometriosis. Reprod Sci. 2008;15(9):906-11.
33. Seeber B, Sammel MD, Fan X, Gerton GL, Shaunik A, Chittams J, Barnhart KT. Panel of markers can accurately predict endometriosis in a subset of patients. Fertil Steril. 2008;89(5):1073-81.
34. John Rendle. Review article—Endometriosis: a radiological review.
35. ESHRE guideline for the diagnosis and treatment of endometriosis (Special Interest Group for Endometriosis and Endometriosis Guideline Development Group. 2007.
36. Endometriosis: diagnosis and management Society of Obstetricians and Gynaecologists of Canada. 2010.
37. Treatment of pelvic pain associated endometriosis. The Practice Committee for the American Society for Reproductive Medicine. 2006.
38. Endometriosis in adolescents (American College of Obstetricians and Gynecologists (ACOG) Committee on Adolescent Health Care – 2005).
39. Ametzazurra A, Matorras R, Garcí´a-Velasco JA, Prieto B, et al. Endometrial fluid is a specific and non-invasive biological sample for protein biomarker identification in endometriosis. Human Reproduction. 2009;24(4):954–65.
40. Cleophas M. Kyama, Attila Mihalyi, Olivier Gevaert, et al. Evaluation of endometrial biomarkers for semi-invasive diagnosis of endometriosis. Fertility and Sterility. 2011;95(4).

Ovarian Endometrioma: Diagnosis and Management

◀ Ramesh B, Sandip Datta Roy

⊃ INTRODUCTION

Endometriosis is a chronic and usually a progressive, painful disorder occurring almost exclusively in women of the reproductive age. The prevalence of endometriosis among asymptomatic women ranges from 2 to 22%,[1] and in women with dysmenorrhea, the incidence is about 40 to 60%.[1] The incidence among the infertile women range between 20 to 50%,[2] and approximately 17 to 44% women with endometriosis have ovarian endometriomas.[3,4] Ovaries are the most frequent site of endometriosis. When ovaries are involved, they become enlarged and cystic, filled with chocolate colored fluid and known as the chocolate cysts or endometriomas. Ovarian endometriomas are a common manifestation of pelvic endometriosis,[5] and most of these patients complain of pain and/or infertility. Endometriomas account for 35% of benign ovarian cysts and associated with organic type of pain such as chronic pelvic pain and dyspareunia.[6] Diagnosing the condition can be difficult at times because the common presenting symptoms, such as pain and infertility, have numerous etiologies and the clinical features may be confused with many other disorders. There is general agreement that laparoscopic conservative surgery is the treatment of choice for ovarian endometrioma, either by cystectomy or by fenestration and coagulation. Surgical treatment is effective in removing the disease and relieving the associated pain symptoms. Laparoscopic cystectomy[7,8] is currently the preferred surgical approach for removal of ovarian endometriomas, because stripping of the cyst wall is associated with a lower risk of recurrence than other procedures,[9] and a better postsurgical spontaneous conception rate than fenestration and coagulation. The available evidence suggest that only medical treatment of endometrioma is inadequate.[10,11]

⊃ PATHOGENESIS OF OVARIAN ENDOMETRIOMAS

The pathogenesis of typical ovarian endometriosis is still a source of controversy. Endometrioma is an ovarian pseudocyst arising from growth of ectopic endometrial tissue, which progressively invaginates the ovarian cortex. Ovarian endometriomas are predominantly hemorrhagic lesions. They results from the implantation of ectopic endometrium on ovarian surface and subsequent invagination and invasion of the endometrium into the ovarian cortex.[12] The cytology of ovarian endometrioma reveals the presence of glandular and flattened endometrial epithelium, endometrial stroma and hemosiderin-laden macrophages.[13] They are probably formed by implantation of viable endometrial tissue on the ovarian surface from retrograde menstrual flow.[14] Hughesdon observed that majority of the ovarian endometriomas develop as a result of progressive invagination of the ovarian cortex due to accumulation of the menstrual blood and debris from the shedding and bleeding of active implants on ovarian surface.[15] Large endometrioma may also develop as a result of the secondary involvement of functional ovarian cysts in the process of endometriosis.[13] Donnez, et al have proposed a different hypothesis on the development of ovarian endometriosis on the basis of celomic metaplasia of the invaginated epithelial inclusions.[16] This hypothesis is based on the metaplastic potential of the pelvic mesothelium. Intraovarian endometriosis or endometrioma are the consequence of metaplasia of invaginated mesothelial inclusions. The cyst contents of endometriomas contain high concentrations of iron and hemosiderin, presumably from chronic bleeding into the cyst, possibly at the time of menstruation. Ovarian endometriomas are frequently observed on the left side and this is probably related to decreased peritoneal fluid movement on the left side of the pelvis due to the presence of sigmoid colon.[17] In majority of the cases, they are monolateral. Both gonads are affected only in 19 to 28% of cases.[18]

⮑ CLINICAL PRESENTATION AND DIAGNOSIS OF ENDOMETRIOMA

Patients with ovarian endometriomas can present with infertility alone or infertility associated with chronic pelvic pain.[19] The clinical presentation of endometriosis does not always correlate with the severity of disease and impact on the physical, mental and social well-being of both symptomatic and asymptomatic women. Majority of patients with endometrioma have pelvic pain, infertility or dyspareunia, either alone or a combination of all these symptoms. Pelvic pain usually occurs during or just before menstruation and lessens after menstruation. Some patients experience painful sexual intercourse or cramping during intercourse when the endometrioma is big and adherent to the pouch of Douglas. The pain intensity can change from month to month, and vary greatly among women. Some women experience progressive worsening of symptoms, while others can have resolution of pain without treatment.

Endometriosis is a recognized cause of infertility and about 30 to 50% women with endometriosis complains of infertility. Both anatomical and hormonal factors are thought to be responsible for infertility.

Ureteral obstruction and hydronephrosis can result from endometrial implants on the ureter or mass effect from an endometrioma. Rupture or torsion of an ovarian endometrioma may present as an acute abdomen.

When the endometrioma is big, a pelvic examination may reveal the presence of an adnexal mass. Clinical history and pelvic examination may not always correlate with the clinical diagnosis. Many a times, endometriomas are diagnosed during evaluation for infertility.

Imaging studies are an integral part for the evaluation of any adnexal mass. Pelvic ultrasonography, computed tomography (CT) scanning, and magnetic resonance imaging (MRI) are useful in the case of advanced disease with endometrial cyst formation or severe anatomic distortion. Endometriomas can be assessed by either transvaginal ultrasonography or endorectal ultra-sonography. The ultrasonographic features of endometriomas vary from simple cysts to complex cysts with internal echoes to solid masses, usually devoid of vascularity. Transvaginal ultrasonography is a useful method of identifying the classic chocolate cyst of the ovary. The typical appearance is that of a cyst containing low-level homogenous internal echoes **(Fig. 4.1)** consistent with old blood.[20] Punctuate echogenecities **(Fig. 4.2)** may be present in the cyst wall and increase the diagnostic confidence. Ultrasound may not differentiate an endometrioma from hemorrhagic cysts, tubo-ovarian abscess and occasionally, cystadenomas. However, features of malignancy such as thick septae and solid areas can be detected by ultrasound.

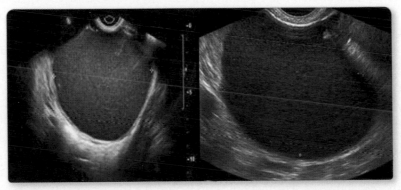

Figure 4.1: Typical endometrioma with low level homogenous internal echos

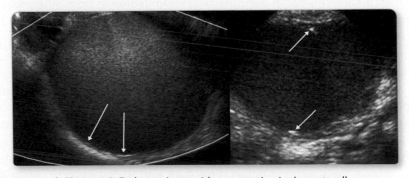

Figure 4.2: Endometrioma with punctuation in the cyst wall

Histopathology is required to make a definitive diagnosis of endometrioma. However, a clinical diagnosis can often be made with a high degree of certainty in a woman with histologically confirmed endometriosis and an adnexal mass, since 50% of women with endometriosis develop endometriomas, which are often bilateral.[21] Ultrasound is useful for supporting the clinical diagnosis of endometrioma, but of limited value for diagnosis or determining extent of endometriosis at other sites since it lacks adequate resolution for visualizing adhesions and superficial peritoneal and ovarian implants. However, when there are sonographic signs suggestive of endometriomas, it is likely that moderate to severe endometriosis is present. Therefore, if pain is the presenting symptom, extensive surgery may be required for relief of pain.[22] Guerriero and colleagues found that the sensitivity and specificity of endovaginal ultrasonography were 83% and 89%, respectively in differentiating endometriomas from other ovarian cysts.[23] However, ultrasound scanning is not as specific as MRI in the evaluation of endometriosis. Compared with laparoscopy, transvaginal ultrasound (TVS) has limited value in diagnosing peritoneal endometriosis but it is a useful tool both to make and to exclude the diagnosis of an ovarian endometrioma.

Doppler waveform analysis is not helpful in differentiating endometriomas from other masses. Low-resistance waveforms resembling malignancy are commonly encountered in endometriomas.[24]

Using computed tomography (CT) scanning, endometriomas may appear as cystic masses, but their appearance is nonspecific and this imaging modality should not be relied on for diagnosis. Complications of endometriosis, including bowel obstruction and hydronephrosis, may be seen on CT scans.

The appearance of endometriomas on MRI is variable and depends on the concentration of iron and protein in the fluid, products of blood degradation.[25] Most endometriomas have the gross appearance of chocolate cysts, representing highly concentrated blood products. MRI demonstrates these endometriomas as cystic masses with very high signal intensity on T1-weighted images and very low signal intensity on T2-weighted images. In one study, MRI showed a sensitivity of 90 to 92% and a specificity of 91 to 98% for the diagnosis of endometrioma in patients with adnexal masses.[26] Thus, MRI is an accurate technique in distinguishing endometriomas from other masses. MRI is not sensitive for superficial implants; therefore, the modality should not be relied on to rule out endometriosis. At present, there is insufficient evidence to indicate that magnetic resonance imaging (MRI) is a useful test to diagnose or exclude endometriosis compared to laparoscopy.

Laparoscopy is the gold standard for the diagnosis of ovarian endometriomas. Laparoscopy allows direct visualization of endometriotic lesions **(Figs 4.3A and B)**, which can be confirmed by biopsy of the excised tissue. Endometriomas usually contain thick fluid like tar. They are often densely adherent to the peritoneum of the ovarian fossa and the surrounding fibrosis may involve the tubes and bowel **(Figs 4.4A and B)**. Because chocolate like fluid may also be found in other types of ovarian cysts, such as hemorrhagic, corpus luteal or neoplastic cysts, biopsy and preferably removal of the cyst for histological confirmation is recommended if the cyst diameter is > 3 cm. Laparoscopy also allow evaluation of superficial peritoneal and ovarian implants. The sensitivity, specificity and diagnostic accuracy of visual diagnosis of endometriomas during laparoscopy is 97%, 95% and 96% respectively.[27]

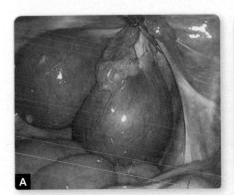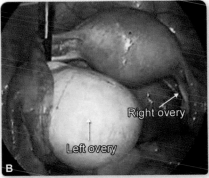

Figures 4.3A and B: (A) Isolated right ovarian endometrioma, (B) Big left ovarian endometrioma

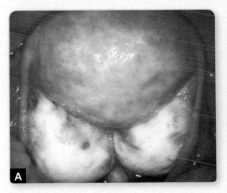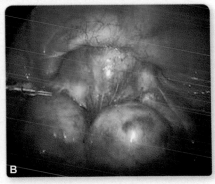

Figures 4.4A and B: (A) Bilateral endometrioma stuck to posterior, (B) Kissing ovaries: Bilateral big endometrioma

Serum CA-125 levels may be elevated in endometriosis. However, compared to laparoscopy, measuring serum CA-125 levels has no value as a diagnostic tool (The ESHRE Guideline on Endometriosis, 2008).

⊃ MANAGEMENT OF ENDOMETRIOMA

Management of endometrioma depends on several factors such as the extent of the disease, severity of symptoms, patient's age, desire for future fertility and whether it is a primary disease or a recurrent endometrioma. Treatment options for pain and infertility with endometriosis include medical and surgical interventions. Treatment of endometrioma is challenged by a high rate of recurrence. Management is more complicated in the setting of infertility and especially before assisted reproductive techniques. The evidence suggests that only medical treatment of endometrioma is inadequate.[28,29] Moreover, ultrasound-guided aspiration is reported to be associated with a high rate of recurrences and complications. Hence, it should be reserved for use in case of postsurgical recurrence or before assisted reproductive technology.[29-31] On the basis of the above considerations, the best surgical approach should be chosen to completely remove all the visible disease, thereby decreasing the risk of recurrence (or possibly persistence) that can result in repetitive surgeries that characterize endometriosis.

⮕ SURGICAL TREATMENT OF ENDOMETRIOMA

Laparoscopic surgery has become a standard in the conservative treatment of ovarian endometriomas. Surgical approaches to relieve endometriosis-related pain are warranted as the first-line treatment for women with pain symptoms who desire to become pregnant as soon as possible or it may be initiated after failed medical therapy.[32] Surgery is also more effective in reducing pain in patients with more advanced endometriosis. There are certain principles that must be followed while managing endometriosis surgically. Malignancy must be ruled out although the incidence is very low (approximately 0.8%).[33] All the active endometrial implants should be removed. Care should be taken to minimize damage to normal ovarian cortex in order to prevent follicular depletion. Adhesions involving the ovary and pelvis should be lysed and measures should be taken to minimize postoperative adhesion formation.

Endometriotic cyst should be treated only in cases of pain and infertility and also, in asymptomatic patients if the cyst diameter is more than 4 cm.[34] The best form of surgical treatment of endometrioma was debated for a long time. Various modalities of conservative laparoscopic surgeries for endometrioma have been described in literature. Basically there are two different techniques to treat endometrioma: fenestration and coagulation of the cyst wall and cystectomy or stripping of the cyst wall. The best surgical treatment for pain, recurrence and infertility associated with endometroma is laparoscopic cystectomy, i.e. excision of the cyst wall.[35] Laparoscopic cystectomy has been considered as the method of choice for the treatment of endometriomas.[36] Although the efficacy of cystectomy and fenestration and cyst wall coagulation is still debated, we perform both the techniques depending on various factors such as the mean diameter of the cyst, feasibility of excision, patient's age and symptoms, and the markers of ovarian reserve, etc.

Surgical Approach

Several non-randomized studies comparing laparotomy with laparoscopic approach to endometrioma have shown that results are similar in terms of pregnancy rates, monthly fecundity, and cyst recurrence rates.[37,38] However, laparoscopy offers the benefits magnification and illumination, less analgesic requirement, shorter postoperative recovery and earlier discharge.[39] Therefore, laparoscopy is considered the best surgical approach for ovarian endometriotic cysts.

Laparoscopic Technique

The patient is placed in modified dorsolithotomy position under general anesthesia and a 10 mm umbilical port is inserted for the laparoscope. Two 5 mm lower abdominal accessory trocars are inserted lateral to the inferior epigastric artery under direct vision. We use 5 mm scissors, atraumatic graspers and toothed graspers for the procedure. Hemostasis can be achieved with bipolar coagulation. Irrigation is done with normal saline. The procedure begins with the inspection of pelvis, pelvic organs, pelvic peritoneum and release of adhesion. The ovary with the cyst is mobilized with 5 mm atraumatic graspers. The ovary may be adherent to lateral pelvic wall, posterior uterine wall and the posterior leaf of the broad ligament or the Fallopian tubes **(Fig. 4.5)**. All the adhesions are carefully removed using sharp dissection with scissors and the ovary is completely mobilized. If the ovary is adherent to the ovarian fossa, care must be taken to avoid ureteric injury while releasing such adhesions.

The next step is puncture and drainage of the endometrioma cavity. The endometrioma can be punctured with the trocar **(Fig. 4.6)** or a small cortical incision can be made with a scissors. Another way is to make a circular incision on the surface of the ovary. Before making the incision, we often infiltrate 20 to 40 ml diluted vasopressin (10 units in 100 ml normal saline) between the ovarian cortex and the cyst wall **(Fig. 4.7)**. It can be done easily with a laparoscopic needle used for vasopressin infiltration during myomectomy. This helps to identify the plane of cleavage between the cyst wall and normal ovarian tissue, thereby making the cystectomy easy and, also reduces the blood loss while stripping the cyst wall. Big cyst cavity can be decompressed by suction drainage. The endometrioma may rupture during manipulation. The content of the endometrioma is carefully aspirated with the suction-irrigator probe and

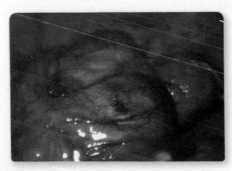

Figure 4.5: Huge left ovarian endometrioma adherent to tube and pelvic sidewall

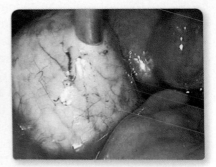

Figure 4.6: Drainage of endometrioma before cystectomy

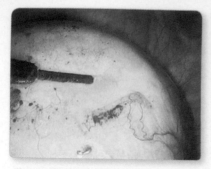

Figure 4.7: Vasopressin infiltration into the cyst wall

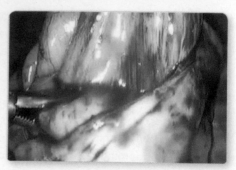

Figure 4.8: Separating the cyst wall from the normal ovarian cortex

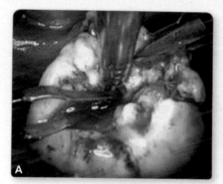

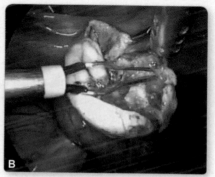

Figures 4.9A and B: Fulguration of cyst wall

the cyst cavity is repeatedly irrigated and aspirated. The inner aspect of the cyst wall is thoroughly inspected for any vegetation and neovascularization that would alert the surgeon to suspect a neoplastic pathology. After identifying the proper plane of cleavage between the cyst wall and the ovarian tissue, the cyst wall and the ovarian cortex is grasped with two 5 mm toothed forceps **(Fig. 4.8)**. Gentle traction and counter traction is applied in opposite directions and the inner lining of the cyst is stripped off the normal ovarian tissue. Excision of the cyst wall of an endometrioma may be difficult at times due to invagination and fibrosis of the cortex. Any residual cyst capsule should be destroyed using monopolar or bipolar thermal energy. When the cyst is < 3 cm in diameter or when it not possible to do a cystectomy due to dense adhesion of fibrosis, the cyst is opened, cyst cavity thoroughly irrigated and the inner wall of the cyst is ablated **(Figs 4.9A and B)**.

After the cyst wall is stripped off, the raw areas in ovarian bed is thoroughly washed to carefully visualize any bleeding points. Hemostasis can be easily achieved by brief application of bipolar graspers to spray coagulate the oozing areas in the ovarian bed. The bleeding can also be controlled by applying pressure with an atraumatic grasper or with application of fibrin glue to approximate the ovarian cortex. After cystectomy, the remaining ovarian tissue is left alone without suturing. Reconstruction with suturing may be required in cases of a big cyst. Fine sutures like 4-0 PDS or vicryl can be used for intraovarian suturing in order to reduce the risk of postoperative adhesion formation around the ovaries, which can further lower the fertility potential and can cause pelvic pain. Adhesion preventing agents like oxydized regenerated cellulose (Interceed) and 4% icodextrin (Adept) can be used to limit postoperative adhesion formation.

The last step is the removal of the excised cyst wall. One of the 5 mm lateral trocars can be converted to a 10 mm trocar and the cyst wall can be removed using a 10 mm claw forceps. Alternatively, a 5 mm laparoscope can be inserted through one of the 5 mm lateral ports and the cyst wall can be removed through the primary 10 mm umbilical port. When cyst wall is voluminous and difficult to remove through the 10 mm trocar, an endobag can be used for retrieval of the tissues. A thorough washing of all the operated areas with normal saline or Ringer lactate is done and all the bleeding points are cauterized to achieve complete hemostasis. The cyst wall is sent for histopathological examination or a biopsy is taken when fenestration and coagulation of the endometrioma is performed.

Complications and Safety Aspects

Complications associated with ovarian endometrioma surgery include premature ovarian failure and postsurgery adhesion formation leading to infertility and chronic pelvic pain. The following strategies can make an ovarian endometrioma surgery safe:

- Keep the ureters under observation when releasing the ovaries from the ovarian fossa
- Identify the right plane before commencing cystectomy as the absence of a clear plane of cleavage between the cyst wall and ovarian tissue could result in unintentional removal of the ovarian cortex and loss of follicles with potential reduction in follicular reserve.[34] Identification of the correct plane may be aided by the use of:
  1. Circular excision and subsequent stripping seem to be more easily performed than direct stripping, although operative times were comparable for both the techniques in literature.[40]
  2. Chemical mucolytic agent "Mesna" (sodium-2-mercaptoethanesulfonate) when applied to surgical planes dissolves the surgical bonds and highlights the anatomical planes, thus enabling easy detachment of tissues.[41] It is directly applied onto the cyst wall drop by drop with a laparoscopic needle with simultaneously exerted progressive and gentle traction on the cyst.
  3. Dilute vasopressin infiltration beneath the capsule before cystectomy.[42]
- Avoid excessive coagulation near the ovarian hilum to avoid compromising ovarian blood supply, thereby reducing chances of premature ovarian failure

❖ Avoid excessive traction on endometrioma capsule near the hilum to avoid hilar vessel tearing

❖ Avoid spillage of the endometriotic tissue in the peritoneal cavity or port site to prevent implantation and growth of endometriotic tissue. Use endobag to retrieve specimens to prevent port site endometriosis

❖ Adhesion barriers are useful in the laparoscopic treatment of endometriosis. Interceed which is oxidized regenerated cellulose has been found to significantly reduce adhesion reformation.[43] Adept (4% icodextrin) is a colorless, nonviscous and iso-osmolar liquid instilled intraperitoneally at the conclusion of surgery, is completely absorbed by 4 days. Adept significantly reduces adhesion scores in laparoscopic treatment of endometriosis.[44] The benefit in adhesion prevention was more pronounced in patients with endometriosis and infertility. It is considered safe, although there was an increased incidence of transient labial edema

❖ When appropriate surgical techniques are applied, small vessels may be identified and selective hemostasis can be accomplished reducing the potential damage to the ovarian parenchyma to a minimum

❖ In case of plurioperated ovaries, when follicular reserve is supposed to be already impaired, this potential risk should be carefully discussed with the patient and be an integral part of the informed consent before surgery.

Role of Adjunctive Surgical Procedures

Laparoscopic uterosacral nerve ablation (LUNA) and presacral neurectomy (LPSN) is sometimes performed along with excisional and ablative procedures to relieve endometriosis-related pelvic pain. LUNA destroys the efferent nerve fibers that travel along the uterosacral ligaments whereas LPSN disrupts the sympathetic pathways from the uterus. There is no evidence that laparoscopic uterine nerve ablation is necessary when ablating endometriotic lesions[45] and laparoscopic uterine nerve ablation by itself has no effect on dysmenorrhea associated with endometriosis.[46] In cases that have failed to respond to conservative laparoscopic surgery, there may be a role for presacral neurectomy, especially in severe dysmenorrhea, although the evidence is inconclusive.[46]

Hormonal Treatment before and after Surgery

Although hormonal therapy prior to surgery improves the revised American Fertility Society classification system (rAFS) scores, there is insufficient evidence of any effect on outcome measures such as pain relief to justify its usage.[47] Compared with surgery alone or surgery plus placebo, postoperative hormonal treatment does not produce a significant reduction in pain recurrence at 12 or 24 months and has no effect on disease recurrence.[47] In a small randomized controlled trial, the LNG-IUS, inserted after laparoscopic surgery for endometriosis associated pain, significantly reduced the risk of recurrent moderate–severe dysmenorrhea at 1 year follow-up.[48] Batioglu et al in a small randomized study found that drainage of the endometriotic cyst followed by GnRH agonist for 6 months was more effective in reducing r-ASRM scores for the endometrial cysts compared with GnRH agonist alone. However, there was no difference in pregnancy rate between the two groups.[49]

Management of Endometrioma in Women with Pelvic Pain

The relationship between chronic pelvic pain symptoms and endometrioma is not very clear. In the majority of cases, it is not possible to relate the pain symptoms to endometrioma *per se* but to the periovarian adhesions or deeply infiltrating endometriosis, which should be treated simultaneously.[50]

Medical treatment is generally effective in relieving the endometriosis related pain. But the painful symptoms usually recur after discontinuation of medical treatment. Studies have shown reduction in the size of small endometriomas after ovarian suppression with danazol or GnRH agonist but large endometriomas do not resolve completely. The decrease in the size of endometrioma varied from 14 to 89% with a mean of 51%.[51] There are no published studies directly investigating the effect of medical treatment, including hormonal suppression on pelvic pain in women with endometrioma. Medical treatment can be offered to women with small symptomatic endometriomas, particularly for those women who wish to avoid surgery.

Surgical treatment of endometrioma is widely accepted as the first line management of symptomatic endometriomas, particularly for women who have completed their family. Surgical treatment include drainage with or without sclerotherapy, drainage with ablation of the cyst wall, drainage and stripping of the cyst wall (ovarian cystectomy) and radical treatment in the form of hysterectomy with or without oophorectomy. Uncontrolled studies reported significant relief of pain in a large proportion of cases after surgical treatment of endometrioma.[52] Large endometriomas may be more susceptible to infection or rupture and should ideally be treated surgically. Excision of endometrioma involves drainage followed by stripping of the cyst wall. Excisional surgery offers advantage over drainage and ablation with respect to the recurrence of endometrioma and the symptoms of dysmenorrhea, deep dyspareunia and non-menstrual pelvic pain.

Laparoscopic or transvaginal ultrasound guided drainage of endometrioma is associated with a high and rapid recurrence rate and is rarely effective in alleviating the patient's symptoms.[53] The administration of GnRH agonist for 3 months after drainage of endometrioma may reduce the revised American Fertility Society grading score for endometriosis by 20% and the mean cyst diameter by 52%.[54] This approach may be useful in women who are at high-risk of surgical complications such as those with a history of previous multiple surgery or those with frozen pelvis.

There is not enough evidence to support the use of hormonal suppression prior to surgical treatment of endometriosis or endometrioma. Although pre-operative hormonal therapy appears to reduce the size of endometrioma, it may induce fibrosis of the capsule, thus increasing the difficulty in stripping the cyst wall without affecting the loss of ovarian follicles.[55]

The evidence regarding the use of COC after surgical treatment of endometriosis or endometrioma is conflicting. Postoperative treatment with a COC has not been shown to be effective after surgical treatment of endometriosis.[56] A recent retrospective study, however, reported a lower recurrence rate in women who used the COC postoperatively.[57] The recurrence rate appeared to be related to the duration of COC use, being lower in women who continued the COC for 24 months than in women who discontinued the COC before the end of the study or those who never used the COC postoperatively. A recent RCT has also found lower recurrence with the use of postoperative COC either cyclically or continuously.[58] However, some authors did not find a benefit from postoperative use of COC in terms of recurrence of endometrioma or moderate-to-severe pain or in the mean time to recurrence of symptoms or endometriomas between the study and the control group.[59]

Hysterectomy with or without salpingo-oophorectomy may be justified in women with advanced endometriosis who do not wish to preserve their fertility. The lowest rates of reoperation for symptomatic endometriosis were in those women who had hysterectomy and bilateral oophorectomy as a primary procedure.[60] However, the disadvantages of oophorectomy should be discussed with the patient.

➲ OOPHORECTOMY FOR ENDOMETRIOMA

Oophorectomy may be considered in women who have significant pain and symptoms despite conservative treatment, do not desire future pregnancies and have severe disease, or are undergoing hysterectomy because of other pelvic conditions, such as fibroids or menorrhagia.[61] Oophorectomy may also be required in case of torsion of endometrioma with gangrene, ovarian abscess with damage to ovarian parenchyma and as a part of hysterectomy with BSO in perimenopausal women. Oophorectomy induces menopause and results in regression of endometriotic lesions. However, the adverse effects related to oophorectomy should be thoroughly informed to the patient before proceeding with such procedures. Since oophorectomy is associated with other significant disadvantages in terms of earlier menopause, hysterectomy with ovarian conservation should be considered for advanced endometriosis in women younger than 40 years.[62]

➲ OVARIAN ENDOMETRIOMA: EFFECT ON FERTILITY AND ITS MANAGEMENT

The specific role of the endometriomas over the reduction of fertility potential remains controversial. Vascular compression is markedly observed in compromised gonads and studies have already demonstrated that 17 to 44%

of the patients with endometriosis related infertility present with ovarian endometriotic cysts. A large endometrioma may replace most of the normal ovarian tissue. Presence of peritubal and periovarian adhesions may distort the pelvic anatomy. Follicular defects like abnormal follicular growth, decreased follicular size and shortened follicular phase are observed in women with mild endometriosis. Impaired ovarian function, pituitary ovarian dysfunction, granulosa cell impairment and uterine function impact on oocyte quality and embryo quality, resulting in ovulatory, fertilization and implantation disorders. It has also been reported that endometriomas may affect the hormonal response to ovarian stimulation regimens with a trend towards fewer oocytes retrieved and a significant reduction in the number of preovulatory follicles.[63] Compromised follicular development and poor embryo quality have been reported to result in impaired fertility outcomes with ovarian endometrioma. The ovarian endometrioma *per se* or surgical removal of endometrioma can cause reduced ovarian reserve and responsiveness to ovarian stimulation.

There are multiple treatment options available for managing ovarian endometrioma with infertility such as expectant management, ultrasound-guided aspiration, drainage of the endometriotic cyst and vaporization of the cyst wall, ovarian fenestration with bipolar electrocoagulation and laparoscopic cystectomy. However, there is a lack of consensus regarding the ideal surgical technique and also on the benefits and drawbacks of surgery. Some studies have found that surgery adversely affects fertility whereas other studies have reported no effect on fertility outcomes. Meticulous surgical techniques should be utilized to minimize damage to healthy ovarian tissue and avoid compromising the blood supply.

Regarding spontaneous pregnancies and recurrence of the cysts and symptoms, a recent systemic review concluded that laparoscopic cystectomy appears to be the best therapeutic choice if compared with drainage or coagulation.[64] Alborzi, et al prospectively evaluated 52 patients submitted to laparoscopic cystectomy and observed spontaneous pregnancy rates of nearly 60% in the first year after surgery, which were statistically significant when compared with the 23.3% obtained after endometrioma fenestration and coagulation.[65]

Expectant management after surgery, with the aim of achieving spontaneous pregnancy, appears to be a good choice, especially for those patients under 35 years of age. However, patients over 35 years or presenting with signs of impaired ovarian function may not be encouraged to decide on expectant management, as they usually present a lower ovarian response. In these cases, ART may be considered as the first-choice treatment, being the laparoscopic procedure dispensable, unless there is no transvaginal access to the ovarian follicles for oocyte pickup.

Therapeutic choice for infertile patients with endometriomas remains a great challenge in the assisted reproduction scenario. There are no randomized controlled trials comparing laparoscopic excision with no treatment before IVF. However, laparoscopic ovarian cystectomy is recommended if an ovarian endometrioma ≥ 4 cm in diameter is present to confirm the diagnosis histologically; reduce the risk of recurrence; improve access to follicles, and possibly improve ovarian response and prevent endometriosis progression. The woman should be counselled regarding the risks of reduced ovarian function after surgery[66,67] and the loss of the ovary. The decision should be reconsidered if she has had previous ovarian surgery (RCOG GTG 24).

Regarding ART results after endometrioma excision, Garcia-Velasco et al retrospectively evaluated 189 women who had undergone IVF treatment following laparoscopic approach to excise lesions and observed no differences between the groups, whatever variety analyzed. They obtained 25.4% of pregnancies among operated women and 22.7% among patients with intact cysts, with no statistical significance, and concluded that no additional benefits were provided by cystectomy.[68] It is possible that excision at cystectomy might negatively affect the success of COH by removing the normal ovarian tissue.[69,70] Accidental removal of a consistent amount of ovarian tissue during cystectomy and the damage inflicted by both surgery-related local inflammation and electrosurgical coagulation of ovarian stroma and vascularization may add to the problem. However, the mean number of dominant follicles and pregnancy rate do not seem to be affected by cystectomy. Moreover, a recent randomized trial has shown that excision or cystectomy does not negatively affect the pregnancy rates in controlled ovarian hyperstimulation in patients with endometriosis.[71]

Treatment with a GnRH agonist for 3 to 6 months before IVF in women with endometriosis increases the rate of clinical pregnancy.

A Cochrane review identified three randomized controlled trials involving women with endometriosis who were treated with a standard protocol or a GnRH agonist for 3 to 6 months before IVF. The clinical pregnancy rate per woman was significantly higher (OR 4.28, 95% CI 2.00–9.15) in women receiving a GnRH agonist compared with controls.[72] However, the authors of the Cochrane review stressed that the recommendation is based on only one properly randomized study and called for further research, particularly on the mechanism of action.

Management of Endometrioma Prior to IVF

Assisted reproduction is widely used to manage infertility associated with endometriosis. IVF may enhance the low fecundity associated with advanced endometriosis. Various studies have evaluated the success of IVF in patients with endometrioma, and some studies have reported beneficial effects.[73,74] while others have reported poor outcomes.[75-77] There is a lack of consensus in the reported literature on outcomes of assisted reproduction in patients with ovarian endometriomas. There are no studies that have evaluated the effects of endometriomas *per se* on IVF outcomes. All of the studies in the literature have investigated IVF outcomes in patients with resected endometriomas or aspirated endometriomas. Many confounding factors can affect pregnancy outcomes such as the size of the endometrioma, previous medical therapy, prior surgical therapy, the type of surgical procedure, interval between therapy and IVF-embryo transfer, and the experience of the surgeon.

IVF is the mainstay of treatment for endometriosis related infertility and consequently, another topic of debate is whether or not endometriomas should be treated before undergoing IVF. A reduced responsiveness to gonadotropin hyperstimulation, reflecting a certain damage to ovarian reserve, is usually noted even in patients with nonoperated endometrioma undergoing IVF. Randomized trials specifically designed to investigate benefits of surgical treatment with respect to expectant management before IVF-ICSI cycles are currently lacking. Patients with nonoperated unilateral endometrioma undergoing IVF can have a mean reduction of 25% (6% to 44%) in the number of codominant follicles in the affected ovaries with respect to the intact ones. Presence of large and multiple cysts in one ovary can further reduce responsiveness to exogenous gonadotrophins.[78] Primordial follicles can be seen histologically close to the cyst wall, probably due to the technical difficulties encountered in removing the cyst, in more than 50% of the endometriomas removed.[79]

The treatment options for women with endometrioma who are about to undergo IVF treatment include surgery, expectant management and medical treatment. The results of studies that compared surgical treatment with no treatment of endometrioma were conflicting. A systematic review and meta-analysis concluded that surgical treatment of endometrioma has no significant effect on IVF pregnancy rates and ovarian response to stimulation compared with no treatment.[80] Although the majority of the studies have suggested a negative effect of surgery on ovarian response to gonadotrophin stimulation, the retrospective nature and the small sample size lessen the conclusion of these studies. Only one RCT investigating the effect of surgical treatment of endometrioma on IVF showed some evidence of reduced ovarian response after surgical excision of endometrioma compared with drainage at the time of oocyte retrieval as evidenced by longer duration of stimulation, higher dose of gonadotrophins used, lower peak oestradiol concentrations and lower number of oocytes retrieved.[81] However, some authors observe that laparoscopic removal of endometriomas before IVF does not compromise the number or quality of oocytes obtained with COH, but at the same time it does not improve fertility outcomes.[82] Hence, cystectomy may be an option when patient has pelvic pain as an associated symptom with infertility.

In the absence of properly designed and powered RCT, the management of endometrioma prior to IVF remains controversial. An ESHRE-sponsored survey[83] to learn the strategies employed for the management of endometrioma (> 3 cm) prior to IVF found that surgical management was the most common treatment

(82.2%), with drainage and excision of the cyst wall being the preferred surgical approach (78.5%). The situation was different for women with previous ovarian surgery or recurrent endometrioma where surgical treatment was less commonly offered. Expectant management of endometrioma remains a major approach in these patients.

Women with endometrioma may include women with normal or poor ovarian reserve. Those with normal ovarian reserve may benefit from prolonged down regulation protocol based on the evidence that this protocol may improve pregnancy rates in women with endometriosis.[84]

Various treatment protocols have been devised to improve ovarian response and pregnancy outcome in women with predicted poor response to ovarian stimulation. Increasing the dose of gonadotrophins has not shown any benefit.[85] With regard to women who had previous ovarian surgery for endometrioma, implantation and clinical pregnancy rates were higher with the GnRH-agonist protocol than with the GnRH-antagonist protocol (22.6% and 39% versus 15.9% and 27.5%, respectively).[86] Further studies are needed to determine the best protocol for ovarian stimulation in poor-responder women with endometrioma.

There is insufficient evidence to support routine surgical treatment of endometrioma in asymptomatic subfertile women. In line with the ESHRE guidelines, expectant management can be offered if endometrioma is smaller than 4 cm and in cases of recurrent endometrioma. Women should be reassured that IVF does not influence the likelihood of endometriosis recurrence.[87,88]

Women who opt for surgical treatment of endometrioma prior to IVF should be offered ovarian reserve tests before surgery and those with reduced ovarian reserve should be discouraged from undergoing surgical treatment. Women undergoing ovarian surgery should be warned about the possible risk of surgery on ovarian function.

Management of Women with Asymptomatic Endometrioma

While the incidence of endometriosis in asymptomatic women ranges from 2 to 50%, there is no population-based studies reporting on the incidence of asymptomatic endometrioma in the general population. Although endometrioma is commonly associated severe endometriosis, there is no correlation between the stages of endometriosis and the severity of pelvic pain symptoms. Factors such as the size of the cyst, accuracy of diagnosis, patient's age and her wish to preserve fertility and ovarian function should be taken into account while managing these patients. Ultrasound scanning and serum CA-125 may help to identify rare cases of ovarian cancer. However, CA-125 levels may be elevated in patients with endometriosis and endometrioma.[89] Due to the increased risk of ovarian cancer, surgical treatment is usually recommended for women above the age of 40 years and for large endometriomas.[90] Those who opt for expectant management, it is prudent to follow them with annual ultrasound scan and serum CA-125.

⮞ ENDOMETRIOMA EXCISION AND OVARIAN RESERVE

Laparoscopic cystectomy is considered the best treatment in terms of lower recurrence and improved fertility. However, it is recently questioned whether the excision of the endometrioma could decrease the function of the operated ovary and if it could subsequently affect the fertility. Removal of normal ovarian tissue and electrosurgical coagulation during hemostasis could play an important role in terms of damage to ovarian stroma and vascularization. Particular attention must be paid in presence of bilateral endometriotic cysts. In fact, an increase in premature ovarian failure rate was reported when both the ovaries are involved in surgery. When surgically approaching bilateral endometriomas, even when the surgical technique is correct, a risk of ovarian reserve reduction should be seriously taken into account. The postsurgical ovarian failure rate can be as high as 2.4% compared with the 1.1% incidence of premature ovarian failure observed in the general population.[91] Currently, no definitive data clarify whether the damage to the ovarian reserve, observed in patient with endometrioma, is related to the surgical procedure, to the previous presence of the cyst, or both. Excision of bilateral endometriomas may be associated with a significantly lower number of follicles, oocytes retrieved and embryos obtained. IVF-ICSI results may be significantly impaired in this particular group of patients.[92] A recent Italian study has shown that ovarian surgery for bilateral endometrioma influences age at menopause. The mean age at menopause among the operated women is significantly lower than mean age of menopause in a reference population.[93] However, several studies have already evaluated ovarian function after endometrioma excision and demonstrated that there were no significant differences between normal and cystectomized ovaries, with satisfactory pregnancy rates. Loh, et al demonstrated a 73.3% pregnancy rate in up to 42 months after surgery, a quarter of them submitted to IVF.[94] Similarly, other studies obtained equivalent pregnancy rates, from 30.5 to 38% per cycle, between women submitted to laparoscopic cystectomy and tubal infertility control group, after induced ovarian cycles.[95,96] Nevertheless, individualization of each case is the most important aspect of management. Based on the current literature, laparoscopic excision of ovarian endometriomas in infertile patients should be considered a good practice. Cyst recurrences should also be carefully evaluated and successive excisions are strongly discouraged owing to their potential risk of diminishing follicle reserve.

⮞ ULTRASOUND-GUIDED ASPIRATION OF ENDOMETRIOMA

Endometriomas have been reported to have depressive effects of endometriomas on oocyte development.[97] Ultrasound-guided aspiration is an option for managing large ovarian endometriomas before IVF that are unlikely to respond to medical treatment alone.[98] Ultrasound-guided aspiration of ovarian endometriomas was proposed in 1991 as an alternative for patients who decline surgery or in whom surgery is contraindicated.[99] The aspiration of the endometriomas was demonstrated to improve the ovarian response with an increase in number of oocytes available for retrieval.[100] Ultrasound-guided endometrioma aspiration can be done at the beginning of ovarian stimulation. It is a less invasive option but it is associated with a high recurrence rate of 66.6%.[101] The high rates of recurrence following this procedure have led to its restricted use. Acute abdominal pain and infectious complications including ovarian abscess formation have been reported following aspiration of endometriomas. The tissue trauma associated with transvaginal drainage or leakage of cyst contents during aspiration or inadvertent rupture may result in adhesion formation. Hormonal suppression therapy following aspiration may reduce the recurrence rates.

➲ SCLEROTHERAPY FOR ENDOMETRIOMA

Simple aspiration of ovarian endometrioma is associated with a high incidence of recurrence. To reduce recurrence, some investigators have combined aspiration with *in situ* injection of a sclerosing agent, for example, tetracycline (5% tetracycline solution), methotrexate, recombinant interleukin-2, or ethanol (95% ethyl alcohol). Studies have shown that ethanol instillation into the cyst cavity for >10 minutes was most effective at reducing the recurrence rate.[102] It is performed in a manner similar to an ovum pickup procedure in IVF. Under vaginal ultrasonographic guidance, a 16-gauge, 35 cm needle is inserted into the endometrioma and its contents aspirated. The cyst cavity is washed with physiological saline and infused with a volume of 95% ethanol equal to 80% of the aspirated volume. The ethanol is left in the cyst cavity for 10 minutes, and then removed. The cellular mechanisms involved in the sclerotherapy of ovarian cysts are not fully known, but it seems that epithelial cells lining the cyst wall play an essential role. When adequate contact between the sclerosing agent and the cyst wall is achieved, the activation of the coagulation cascade and the production of mediators of inflammation and fibrosis by epithelial lining cells lead to cyst wall adherence. Treatment of ovarian endometriomas by aspiration and sclerotherapy with 95% ethanol is a simple and effective therapy with a relatively low recurrence rate of 13.3%.[103] Although the evidence is insufficient, drainage and sclerotherapy of endometrioma, possibly followed by postoperative ovarian suppression for 3 months, may be valid for women with a history of previous multiple surgery or those with frozen pelvis who wish to preserve their ovaries.

➲ RECURRENT ENDOMETRIOMA AND ITS MANAGEMENT

Surgical treatment of ovarian endometrioma is associated with a high recurrence rate. Busacca, et al observed a cumulative rate of ultrasonographic recurrence of 11.7% and a cumulative rate of a second surgery of 8.2% over 48 months. Ultrasonographic cyst recurrence was associated with pain recurrence in 73% of cases.[104] The stage of the disease and a history of previous surgery for endometriosis are the most important factors associated with recurrence of endometrioma. Higher recurrence rate has also been reported with previous medical treatment and large endometrioma. Coagulation or laser vaporization of endometriomas without excision of the pseudocapsule seems to be associated with a significant increase in risk of cyst recurrence. Recurrence after surgery occurs because of *in situ* regrowth of residual endometriotic lesions or it may be due to residual cells not completely removed during surgery. Recurrence can also be due to growth of microscopic endometriosis undetected at surgery, or the development of de novo lesions, or a combination of these.

The primary goal in the management of recurrent disease is the treatment of pain and/or restoration or preservation of fertility. Medical treatment aims at ovarian suppression with GnRH agonist, combined OCP, LNG-IUS, etc. The decision to reoperate depends less on the endometrioma size than on symptoms, in particular severe pain, and failure of medical treatment. However, such patients are also more likely to have signs of deep nodules and adnexal/bowel adhesions and larger endometriomas on TVS scan, thus predisposing them to require a second procedure.[105]

Postoperative GnRH agonist treatment for 6 months reduces endometriosis associated pain and delays pain recurrence at 12 and 24 months compared with placebo and expectant management.[106] Recently, an updated online version of the ESHRE guidelines mentioned that treatment for 3 months with GnRH agonist may be as effective 6 months in terms of pain relief.[107]

For patients with infertility without pain, the recurrence of endometriomas may be treated with either surgery or ART. The advantage of ART is that it avoids surgery, which is more risky and may further compromise ovarian reserve and function, as suggested by several investigators.[108] The probability of conception after repeat surgery for recurrent endometriosis appears reduced compared with that after primary surgery. The loss of functional ovarian tissue associated with repeat surgery may be clinically significant in patients undergoing fertility therapy. However, loss or diminution of ovarian reserve associated with a second resection of recurrent endometriomas is presently controversial. Some studies suspect a reduced ovarian reserve after second surgery, and some suggest non-surgical treatment of endometriomas especially if the cyst volume is small. Because poor ovarian response is probably not related to the presence of endometriomas alone but to other factors, including surgical trauma, some authors suggest not removing endometriomas before IVF.[109-111] However, some authors have reported that after laparoscopic excision of recurrent ovarian endometriomas, the recurrence of pain and the reproductive outcome are comparable with those found after primary surgery.[112] The IVF results are not impulled by the presence of endometriomas. It is not prudent to reoperate for endometriosis before IVF. In severe stages or in cases of recurrence, a pre-IVF medical treatment with two months GnRH agonist may improve the results. Transvaginal aspiration of cyst before starting the stimulation is another option.

⊃ ENDOMETRIOMA AND OVARIAN CANCER

The risk of ovarian cancer is slightly increased in women with endometrioma.[113] Some endometriosis lesions may predispose to clear cell and endometrioid ovarian cancers. Advancing age and the size of endometriomas were independent predictors of development of ovarian cancer among women with ovarian endometrioma. A cyst diameter more than 9 cm and postmenopausal status were found to be independent risk factors.[113] Local guidelines for the management of suspected ovarian malignancy should be followed in cases of ovarian endometrioma. Ultrasound scanning ± serum CA-125 testing is usually used to try to identify rare instances of ovarian cancer. However, CA-125 levels can be elevated in the presence of endometriomas.(The ESHRE Guideline on Endometriosis, 2008).

⊃ CONCLUSION

Endometriomas are commonly seen in women of reproductive age who may wish to preserve their ovarian function and/or fertility. The treatment options for symptomatic endometrioma should be individualized depending on the patient's age and her desire for fertility, previous surgery and associated risks, long-term effects of medical therapy and last but not the least, patient's preference. Medical treatment should be offered to symptomatic women with small endometrioma who wish to avoid surgery. Conservative surgical treatment is generally preferred for premenopausal women who wish to preserve their ovarian function. Radical treatment is best reserved for older women who have completed their family.

Laparoscopic surgery has become the standard of care in the conservative treatment of ovarian endometriomas. However, the best surgical technique for the treatment of endometriomas is still controversial. Laparoscopic cystectomy is better than drainage and coagulation in reducing pain symptoms, rates of recurrence and it also improves subsequent spontaneous pregnancy rates.

There is increasing concern about removal of normal ovarian tissue during cystectomy that may reduce ovarian follicle reserve. But, based on the current evidence, ovarian cystectomy seems to be the method of choice with a significantly decreased risk of cyst recurrence. In case of assisted reproductive techniques, there is no clear concensus about the best approach for concomitant endometriotic cyst. Laparoscopic excision of ovarian endometrioma prior to IVF does not offer any additional benefit over expectant management in terms of ovarian response to gonadotrophin stimulation or pregnancy outcome. A large, well-designed and adequately powered randomized controlled trial that compares the effects of surgical removal versus expectant management of endometrioma on ovarian function and pregnancy outcomes in women undergoing IVF is warranted. Until then management of endometrioma prior to IVF should be individualized to maximize the chances of success and minimize risks. Postoperative hormonal treatment has no beneficial effect on pregnancy rates after surgery. Compared with surgery alone or surgery plus placebo, postoperative hormonal treatment has no effect on pregnancy rates.[114] All therapeutic options including conservative, medical or surgical treatment as well as the advantages and disadvantages should be properly discussed with the patient. Any decision for surgery should be carefully balanced against the risks in women with prior surgery or those with suboptimal ovarian reserve.

⊃ REFERENCES

1. Farquar CM. Endometriosis. BMJ. 2000;320:1449-52.
2. Kuligowska E, Deeds L, Lu K. Pelvic pain: Overlooked and underdiagnosed gynecologic conditions. Radiographics. 2005;25:3-20.
3. Jetkins S, Olive DL, Haney AF. Endometriosis: Pathogenic implications of the anatomic distribution. Obstet Gynecol. 1986;67:335-8.
4. Redwine DB. Ovarian endometriosis: A marker for extensive pelvic and intestinal disease. Fertil Steril. 1999;72:310315.
5. Gruppo italiano per lo studio dell' endometriosis. Endometriosis: Prevalence and anatomical distribution of endometriosis in women with selected gynecological conditions; results from a multicentric Italian study. Hum Reprod.1994;9:1158-62.
6. Vercillini P. Endometriosis: What pain it is. Semin Reprod Endocrin. 1997;15:251-6.
7. Crosignani PG, Vercellini P, Biffignandi F, Costantini W, Cortesi I, Imparato E. Laparoscopy versus laparotomy in conservative surgical treatment for severe endometriosis. Fertil steril 1996;66:706-11.
8. Abbott J, Hawe J, Hunter D, Holmes M, Finn P, Garry R. Laparoscopic excision of endometriosis: a randomized, placebo-controlled trial. Fertil steril 2004;82:878-84.
9. Garry R. The effectiveness of laparoscopic excision of endometriosis. Curr Opin Obstet Gynecol 2004;16:299-303.
10. Bateman BG, Kolp LA, Mills S. Endoscopic versus laparotomy management of endometriomas. Fertil steril 1994;62:690-95.
11. Catalano GF, Marana R, Caruana p, et al. Laparoscopy versus microsurgery via laparotomy for excision of ovarian cysts in patients with moderate or severe endometriosis. J Am Assoc Gynecol Laparosc. 1996;3:267-70.
12. Brosens I. Endometriosis and the outcome of In vitro fertilization. Fertil and Steril. 2004; 81:1198–200.
13. Nezhat F, Nezhat C, Allan CJ, et al. Clinical and histologic classification of endometriomas. Implications for a mechanism of pathogenesis. Reprod Med 1992; 37:771-6.
14. Sampson JA. Peritoneal endometriosis due to the menstrual dissemination of endometrial tissue into the peritoneal cavity. Am. J. Obstet. Gynecol. 1927;14:422-69.
15. Hughesdon, PE. The structure of endometrial cysts of the ovary. J. Obstet. Gynecol. Br. Emp. 1957; 44:69-84.

16. Donnez J, M Nisolle, N Gillet, et al. Large ovarian endometriomas. Hum Reprod 1996;11:641-6.
17. Haya Al-Fozan, Togas Tolandi. Left lateral predisposition of endometriosis and endometrioma. Obstet Gynecol. 2003;101:164-6.
18. Vercellini P, Aimi G, De Giorgi O, Maddalena S, Carinelli S, Crosignani PG. Is cystic ovarian endometriosis an asymptomatic disease? Br J Obstet Gynecol. 1998;105:1018-21.
19. Milingos S, Protopapas A, Kallipolitis G, et al. Laparoscopic evaluation of infertile patients with chronic pelvic pain. Reprod BioMed Online. 2006;12:347–53.
20. Asch E, Levine D. Variations in appearance of endometriomas. J Ultrasound Med. 2007;26(8):993-1002.
21. Busacca M, Riparini J, Somigliana E, et al. Postsurgical ovarian failure after laparoscopic excision of bilateral endometriomas. Am J Obstet Gynecol. 2006;195(2):421.
22. Ghezzi F, Raio L, Cromi A, et al. "Kissing ovaries": A sonographic sign of moderate to severe endometriosis. Fertil Steril. 2005;83(1):143
23. Guerriero S, Mais V, Ajossa S, et al. The role of endovaginal ultrasound in differentiating endometriomas from other ovarian cysts. Clin Exp Obstet Gynecol. 1995;22(1):20-2.
24. Alcazar JL, Laparte C, Jurado M, Lopez-Garcia G. The role of transvaginal ultrasonography combined with color velocity imaging and pulsed Doppler in the diagnosis of endometrioma. Fertil Steril. 1997;67(3):487-91.
25. Gougoutas CA, Siegelman ES, Hunt J, et al. Pelvic endometriosis: various manifestations and MR imaging findings. AJR Am J Roentgenol. 2000;175(2):353-8.
26. Togashi K, Nishimura K, Kimura I, et al. Endometrial cysts: diagnosis with MR imaging. Radiology. 1991;180(1):73-78.
27. Vercillini P, Vendola N, Bocciolone L, et al. Reliability of visual diagnosis of ovarian endometriosis. Fertil Steril 1997;67:487-91.
28. Farquhar C, Sutton C. The evidence for the management of endometriosis. Curr Opin Obstet Gynecol. 1998;10:321–32.
29. Chapron C, Vercellini P, Barakat H, et al. Management of ovarian endometriomas. Hum Reprod Update. 2002;8:591–7.
30. Muzii L, Marana R, Caruana P, et al. Laparoscopic findings after transvaginal ultrasound-guided aspiration of ovarian endometriomas. Hum Reprod. 1995;10: 2902–3.
31. Zanetta G, Lissoni A, Dalla Valle C, et al. Ultrasound-guided aspiration of endometriomas: possible applications and limitations. Fertil Steril. 1995;64:709–13.
32. Jacobson TZ, Duffy JM, Barlow D, et al. Cochrane Database Syst Rev. 2009;4:CD001300.
33. Benoit L, Arnould L, Margarot A, et al. Malignant tumours arising in extraovarian endometriosis: Three case reports and review of the literature. Ann Chir 2004; 129(6-7):376-80.
34. Mauro B, Michele V. Endometrioma excision and ovarian reserve: A dangerous Relation. Journal Min Invas Gyne. 2009;19:12-148.
35. Patric Peter Yeung Jr, James Shwayder, Resad P Pasic. Laparoscopic management of endometriosis: Comprehensive review of best evidence. Jour Minim Invas Gyne. 2009;16(3):269-81.
36. Garry R. Laparoscopic excision of endometriosis: The treatment of choice? Br J Obstet Gynaecol. 1997;104:513-5.
37. Sawada T, Satoshi O, kawakami S. Laparoscopic surgery vs laparotomy management for infertile patients with ovarian endometriomas. Gynecol Endosc. 1999;8:7-19.

38. Busaca M, Fedele L, Bianchi S, et al. Surgical treatment of recurrent endometriosis: laparotomy versus laparoscopy. Hum Reprod. 1998;13:2271-4.
39. Maïs V, Ajossa S, Guerriero S, et al. Laparoscopic management of endometriomas: a randomized trial versus laparotomy. J Gynecol surg. 1996;12:41-6.
40. Muzzi L, Bellati F, Palaia I, et al. Laparoscopic stripping of endometriomas: A randomized trial on different surgical techniques. Part I: clinical results. Hum Reprod. 2005;20:1981-6.
41. Benassi L, Benassi G, Kaihura CT, Marconi L, Ricci L, Vadora E. Chemically assisted dissection of tissues in laparoscopic excision of endometriotic cysts. J Am Assoc Gynecol Laparosc. 2003;10:205-9.
42. Sakei A, Matsumoto T, Ikuma K, et al. The vasopressin injection technique for laparoscopic excision of ovarian endometrioma: A technique to reduce the use of coagulation. Mini Invas Gyne. 2010;17(2):176-9.
43. Mais V, Ajossa S, Marongiu D, et al. Reduction of adhesion reformation after laparoscopic endometriosis surgery: a randomized trial with an oxidized regenerated cellulose absorbable barrier. Obstet Gynecol. 1995;86:512-15.
44. Brown CB, Luciano AA, Martin D, et al. Adept Adhesion Reduction Study Group. Adept (4% icodextrin solution) reduces adhesion after laparoscopic surgery adhesolysis: a double blind, randomized controlled study. Fertil Steril. 2007;88: 1413-26.
45. Sutton C, Pooley AS, Jones KD, Dover RW, Haines P. A prospective, randomized, double–blind controlled trial of laparoscopic uterine nerve ablation in the treatment of pelvic pain associated with endometriosis. Gynaecol Endosc 2001;10:217–22.
46. Proctor M, Latthe P, Farquhar C, Khan K, Johnson N, Proctor M. Surgical interruption of pelvic nerve pathways for primary and secondary dysmenorrhoea. Cochrane Database Syst Rev 2005;(4):CD001896.
47. Yap C, Furness S, Farquhar C. Pre and postoperative medical therapy for endometriosis surgery. Cochrane Database Syst Rev 2004;(3):CD003678.
48. Vercellini P, Frontino G, De Giorgi O, Aimi G, Zaina B, Crosignani PG. Comparison of a levonorgestrel–releasing intrauterine device versus expectant management after conservative surgery for symptomatic endometriosis: a pilot study. Fertil Steril. 2003;80:305–9.
49. Batioglu S, Celikkanat H, Ugur M, Mollamahamutoglu L, Yesilyurt H, Kundakci M. The use of GnRH agonists in the treatment of endometriomas with or without drainage. J Pak Med Assoc. 1996;46:30-2.
50. Fauconnier A, Chapron C. Endometriosis and pelvic pain: epidemiological evidence of the relationship and implications. Hum. Reprod. Update 2005; (11): 595–606.
51. Rana N, Thomas S, Rotman C, Dmowski WP. Decrease in the size of ovarian endometriomas during ovarian suppression in stage IV endometriosis. Role of preoperative medical treatment. J Reprod Med 1996;41: 384–32.
52. Jones KD, Sutton C . Patient satisfaction and changes in pain scores after ablative laparoscopic surgery for stage III-IV endometriosis and endometriotic cysts. Fertil Steril. 2003; 79:1086–90.
53. Chan LY, So WW, Lao TT. Rapid recurrence of endometrioma after transvaginal ultrasound-guided aspiration. Eur J Obstet Gynecol Reprod Biol. 2003;15:196–8.
54. Donnez J, Nisolle M, Gillerot S, Anaf V, Clerckx-Braun F, Casanas-Roux F. Ovarian endometrial cysts: the role of gonadotropin-releasing hormone agonist and/or drainage. Ferti Steril. 1994;62: 63–6.
55. Tsujioka, H, Inoue Y, Emoto M, Sadamori R, Shirota K, Hachisuga T, et al. The efficacy of preoperative hormonal therapy before laparoscopic cystectomy of ovarian endometriomas. J Obstet Gynaec Res 2009;35: 782–6.

56. Muzii L, Marana R, Caruana P, Catalano GF, Margutti F, Panici PB. Postoperative administration of monophasic combined oral contraceptives after laparoscopic treatment of ovarian endometriomas: a prospective, randomized trial. Am J Obstet Gynecol 2000; 183: 588–92.

57. Takamura M, Koga K, Osuga Y, Takemaru Y, Hamasoki K, Hirota Y, et al. Postoperative oral contraceptive use reduces the risk of ovarian endometrioma recurrence after laparoscopic excision. Hum. Reprod. 2009;24:3042–8.

58. Seracchioli R, Mabrouk M, Frasca C, Manuzzi L, Montanari G, Keramyda A, et al. Long-term cyclic and continuous oral contraceptive therapy and endometrioma recurrence: a randomized controlled trial. Fertil Steril. 2010;93: 52–6.

59. Sesti F, Capozzolo T, Pietropolli A, Marziali M, Bollea MR, Piccione E. Recurrence rate of endometrioma after laparoscopic cystectomy: a comparative randomized trial between postoperative hormonal suppression treatment or dietary therapy vs. placebo. Eur J Obstet Gynecol Reprod Biol 2009:147: 72–7.

60. Shakiba K, Bena JF, McGill KM, Minger J, Falcone T. Surgical treatment of endometriosis: a 7-year follow-up on the requirement for further surgery. Obstet. Gynecol. 2008;111: 1285–92.

61. Society of obstetricians and gynaecologists of Canada. Endometriosis: Diagnosis and Management. Clinical Practice Guideline no 244. Obste Gynae, Canada. 2010;32:7.

62. Shakiba K, Bena JF, McGill KM, Minger J, Falcone T. Surgical treatment of endometriosis: a 7-year follow-up on the requirement for further surgery. Obstet Gynecol. 2008;111: 1285–92.

63. Al-Azemi M, Bernal AL, Steele J et al. Ovarian response to repeated controlled stimulation in *in vitro* fertilization cycles in patients with ovarian endometriosis. Hum Reprod 2000;15:72–5.

64. Hart R, Hickey M, Maouris P, et al. Excisional surgery versus ablative surgery for ovarian endometriomata: A Cochrane review. Hum Reprod. 2005;20(11):3000-7.

65. Alborzi S, Momtahan M, Parsanezhad ME, et al. A prospective, randomized study comparing laparoscopic ovarian cystectomy versus fenestration and coagulation in patients with endometriomas. Fertil Steril. 2004;82(6):1633-7.

66. Garcia-Velasco JA, Mahutte NG, Corona J, et al. Removal of endometriomas before *in vitro* fertilization does not improve fertility outcomes: a matched, case–control study. Fertil Steril. 2004;81:1194–7.

67. Somigliana E, Ragni G, Benedetti F, et al. Does laparoscopic excision of endo-metriotic ovarian cysts significantly affect ovarian reserve? Insights from IVF cycles. Hum Reprod. 2003;18:2450–3.

68. Garcia-Velasco JA, Mahutte NG, Corona J, et al. Removal of endometriomas before *in vitro* fertilization does not improve fertility outcomes: A matched, case-control study. Fertil Steril. 2004;81(5):1194-7.

69. Ho HY, Lee RK, Hwu YM, Lin MH, Su JT, Tsai YC. Poor response of ovaries with endometrioma previously treated with cystectomy to control ovarian hyperstimulation. J Assst Reprod Genet. 2002;19:507-11.

70. Somigliana E, Ragni G, Benedetti F, Borroni R, Vegett W, Corsignani PG. Does laparoscopic excision of endometriotic ovarian cysts significantly affect ovarian reserve? Insights from IVF cycles. Hum Reprod. 2003;18:2450-3.

71. Alborzi S, Ravanbakhsh R, Parsanezhad E, Alborzi M, Alborzi S, Dehbashi S. A comparison of follicular response of ovaries to ovulation induction after laparoscopic ovarian cystectomy or fenestration and coagulation versus normal ovaries in patient with ovarian endometrioma. Fertil Steril. 2007;88:507-9.

72. Sallam HN, Garcia-Velasco JA, Dias S, Arici A. Long-term pituitary down-regulation before *in vitro* fertilization (IVF) for women with endometriosis. Cochrane Database Syst Rev 2006;(1):CD004635.
73. Tinkanen H, Kujansuu E. *In vitro* fertilization in patients with ovarian endometriomas. Acta Obstetricia et Gynecologica Scandinavica. 2000;79:119–22.
74. Suganuma N, Wakahara Y, Ishida D, et al. Pretreatment for ovarian endometrial cyst before *in vitro* fertilization. Gynec and Obste Investig 2002;54 (Suppl. 1), 36-40; discussion 41-2.
75. Dlugi AM, Loy RA, Dieterle S, et al. The effect of endometriomas on *in vitro* fertilization outcome. J of *In Vitro* Fertil and Embry Trans. 1989; 6:338–41.
76. Yanushpolsky EH, Best CL, Jackson KV, et al. Effects of endometriomas on oocyte quality, embryo quality, and pregnancy rates in *in vitro* fertilization cycles: a prospective, case-controlled study. J Assist Reprod and Genet.1998;15:193–7.
77. Geber S, Ferreira DP, Spyer Prates LF, et al. Effects of previous ovarian surgery for endometriosis on the outcome of assisted reproduction treatment. Reprod BioMed Online . 2002;5:162–6.
78. Somigliana E, Infantino M, Benedetti F, Arnoldi M, Calanna G, Ragni G. The presence of ovarian endometriomas is associated with a reduced responsiveness to gonadotropins. Fertil Steril. 2006;86:192–6.
79. Hachisuga T, Kawarabayashi T. Histopathological analysis of laparoscopically treated ovarian endometriotic cysts with special reference to loss of follicles. Hum Reprod. 2002;17:432–5.
80. Tsoumpou I, Kyrgiou, M, Gelbaya TA. The effect of surgical treatment for endometrioma on *in vitro* fertilization outcomes: a systematic review and meta-analysis. Fertil Steril. 2009; 92:75–87.
81. Demirol A, Guven S, Baykal C, Gurgan, T. Effect of endometrioma cystectomy on IVF outcome: a prospective randomized study. Reprod Biomed Online. 2006;12: 639–43.
82. Garcia-Velasco JA, Mahutte NG, Corona J, et al. Removal of endometriomas before *in vitro* fertilization does not improve fertility outcomes: a matched, case-control study. Fertil Steril. 2004;81:1194–7.
83. Gelbaya TA, Gordts S, D'Hooghe TM, Gergolet M, Nardo LG. Management of endometrioma prior to *in vitro* fertilization: compliance with ESHRE guidelines. Reprod Biomed Online. 2010.
84. Sallam HN, Garcia-Velasco JA, Dias S, Arici A. Long-term pituitary down-regulation before *in vitro* fertilization (IVF) for women with endometriosis. Cochrane Database Syst Rev. 2006: (25): CD004635.
85. Klinkert ER, Broekmans FJM, Looman CWN, Habbema JDF, te Velde ER. Expected poor responders on the basis of an antral follicle count do not benefit from a higher starting dose of gonadotrophins in IVF treatment: A randomized controlled trial. Hum Reprod. 2005;20: 611–5.
86. Pabuccu R, Onalan G, Kaya C. GnRH agonist and antagonist protocols for stage I–II endometriosis and endometrioma in *in vitro* fertilization/intracytoplasmic sperm injection cycles. Fertil Steril. 2007;88: 832–9.
87. Benaglia L, Somigliana E, Vighi V, Nicolosi AE, Iemmello R, Ragni G. Is the dimension of ovarian endometriomas significantly modified by IVF–ICSI cycles? Reprod Biomed Online. 2009;18: 401–6.
88. Benaglia L, Somigliana E, Vercellini P, Benedetti F, Iemmello R, Vighi V. The impact of IVF procedures on endometriosis recurrence. Eur J Obstet Gynecol Reprod Biol. 2010;148: 49–52.

89. Kennedy S, Bergqvist A, Chapron C, et al. ESHRE guideline for the diagnosis and treatment of endometriosis. Hum Reprod. 2005;20:2698-2704.
90. Kobayashi H, Sumimoto K, Kitanaka T, et al. Ovarian endometrioma: risk factors for ovarian cancer development. Eur J Obstet Gynecol Reprod Biol. 2008;138:187-93.
91. Busacca M, Riparini J, Somigliana E, et al. Postsurgical ovarian failure after laparoscopic excision of bilateral endometrioms. Am J Obstet Gynecol. 2006;195:421-5.
92. Somigliana E, Arnoldi M, Benaglia L, et al. IVF-ICSI outcome in in women operated on for bilateral endometriomas. Hum Reprod. 2008;23:1526-30.
93. Coccia ME, Rizzelo F, Mariani G, et al. Ovarian surgery for bilateral endometriomas influences age at menopause. Hum Reprod. 2011;26:3000-7.
94. Loh FH, Tan AT, Ruman J, Ng SC. Ovarian response after laparoscopic ovarian cystectomy for endometriotic cysts in 132 monitored cycles. Fertil. Steril. 1999;72(2): 316-21.
95. Canis M, Pouly JL, Tamburro S, Mage G, Wattiez A, Bruhat MA. Ovarian response during IVF-embryo transfer cycles after laparoscopic ovarian cystectomy for endometriotic cysts of > 3 cm in diameter. Hum. Reprod. 2001;16(12): 2583-6.
96. Marconi G, Vilela M, Quintana R, Sueldo C. Laparoscopic ovarian cystectomy of endometriomas does not affect the ovarian response to gonadotropin stimulation. Fertil. Steril. 2002;78(4): 876-8.
97. Suzuki T, Izumi S, Matsubayashi H, et al. Impact of ovarian endometrioma on oocytes and pregnancy outcome in *in vitro* fertilization. Fertil and Steril. 2005;83: 908–13.
98. Mittal S, Kumar S, Kumar A, et al. Ultrasound guided aspiration of endometrioma: A new therapeutic modality to improve reproductive outcome. Intern J of Gynaec and Obst. 1999;65:17–23.
99. Aboulghar MA, Mansour RT, Serour GI, Rizk B. Ultrasonic transvaginal aspiration of endometriotic cysts: an optional line of treatment in selected cases of endometriosis. Hum Reprod. 1991;6:1408–10.
100. Dicker D, Goldman JA, Feldberg D, et al. Transvaginal ultrasonic needle-guided aspiration of endometriotic cysts before ovulation induction for *in vitro* fertilization. J of *In Vitro* Fertil and Embryo Trans. 1991; 8: 286- 9.
101. Troiano RN, Taylor KJ. Sonographically guided therapeutic aspiration of benign-appearing ovarian cysts and endometriomas. Am J of Roentgen.1998;171:1601–5.
102. Noma J, Yoshida N. Efficacy of ethanol sclerotherapy for ovarian endometriomas. Int J Gynecol Obstet 2001;72:35–9.
103. Hsieh CL, Shiau CS, Lo LM, et al. Effectiveness of ultrasound-guided aspiration and sclerotherapy with 95% ethanol for treatment of recurrent ovarian endometriomas. Fertil and Steril. 2009;91:2709-13.
104. Busacca M, Marana R, Caruana P, Candianl M, Muzii L, Calia C. Recurrence of ovarian endometrioma after laparoscopic excision. Am J Obstet Gynecol. 1999;180: 519–23.
105. Exacoustos C, Zupi E, Amadio A, et al. Recurrence of endometriomas after laparoscopic removal: Sonographic and clinical follow-up and indication for second surgery. J Mini Invas Gynec. 2006;13:281–8.
106. Kennedy S, Bergqvist A, Chapron C, et al. ESHRE guidelines for the diagnosis and treatment of endometriosis. Hum Reprod. 2005;20:2698-704.
107. Hornstein MD, Yuzpe AA, Burry KA, et al. Prospective randomized double-blind trial of 3 versus 6 months of nafarelin therapy for endometriosis related pelvic pain. Fertil Steril. 1995;63:955-62.
108. Loh FH, Tan AT, Kumar J, Ng SC. Ovarian response after laparoscopic ovarian cystectomy for endometriotic cysts in 132 monitored cycles. Fertil Steril. 1999;72:316–21.

109. Garcia-Velasco JA, Mahutte NG, Corona J, et al. Removal of endometriomas before *in vitro* fertilization does not improve fertility outcomes: a matched case-control study. Fertil Steril. 2004;81:1194–7.
110. Pabuccu R, Onalan G, Goktolga U, Kucuk T, Orhon E, Ceyhan T. Aspiration of ovarian endometriomas before intracytoplasmic sperm injection. Fertil Steril. 2004;82: 705–11.
111. Wong BC, Gillman NC, Oehninger S, Gibbons WE, Stadtmauer LA. Results of *in vitro* fertilization in patients with endometriomas: Is surgical removal beneficial? Am J Obstet Gynecol. 2004;19:597–607.
112. Fedele L, Bianchi S, Zanconato G, et al. Laparoscopic excision of recurrent endometriomas: Long-term outcome and comparision with primary surgery. Fertil Steril. 2006;85(3):694-9.
113. Kobayashi H, Sumimoto K, Kitanaka T, et al. Ovarian endometrioma: Risks factors of ovarian cancer development. Eur J Obstet Gynecol Reprod Biol 2008;138:187–93.
114. Yap C, Furness S, Farquhar C, Pre and postoperative medical therapy for endometriosis surgery. Cochrane Database Syst Rev 2004,(3):CD003678.

Endometriosis and Infertility

◀ Pratap Kumar, Prashant Joshi

Endometriosis is an enigmatic disease which affects nearly 5 to 10% of reproductive aged women causing pain and infertility. Endometriosis is present in 25 to 40% of women with infertility and 30 to 50% of women with endometriosis are infertile.[1] The monthly fecundity rate of women with endometriosis is 0.02 to 0.10 compared to 0.15 to 0.20 in fertile women.[2] Though the association between endometriosis and infertility is generally accepted, a casual relation has not yet been established and the mechanism of action resulting in decreased cycle fecundity remains unproven. Although severe endometriosis distorts pelvic anatomy and reduces fertility by mechanical means, mild endometriosis is commonly found in women with infertility. However, the effect of endometriosis on fertility appears to be dose dependent and more severe the disease more profound the effect seems. Expectant management alone allows half the patients with mild disease to conceive, whereas only a quarter with moderate disease and only a few with severe disease are successful.[3]

➲ PATHOGENESIS

Infertility caused by endometriosis is difficult to explain in mild disease but in severe disease mechanical distortions caused by adhesions, endometriomas and repeated surgeries could be the explanation **(Fig. 5.1)**.

In mild disease several mechanisms have been hypothesized. Altered immunological and the resulting inflammation could cause infertility in a number of ways. Abnormal cytokines in the peritoneal fluid may cause sperm immobilization or interfere with sperm-oocyte interaction or decrease the oocyte quality and embryo quality.

The ovarian reserve may be affected in women with endometriosis as evidenced by decreased anti Mullerian hormone in women with endometriosis. Furthermore, endometriomas and surgical treatment involving ovaries can also cause a decrease in ovarian reserve by causing a reduction in functional ovarian tissue.

- ❖ Biologic mechanisms that may link endometriosis and infertility
    - – Distorted pelvic anatomy
        - • Adhesions impair oocyte release and/or ovum pickup

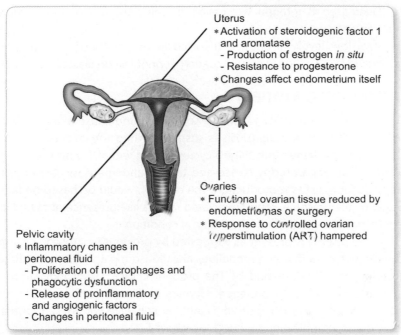

Figure 5.1: Pathogenesis of infertility associated with endometriosis

- Altered peritoneal function
  - Women with endometriosis are noted to have following
    - Increased volume peritoneal fluid
    - Increased peritoneal fluid concentration of the following
      * Activated macrophages
      * Prostaglandins
      * Interleukin-1
      * Tumor necrosis factor
      * Proteases
    - Peritoneal fluid contains ovum capture inhibitor (prevents normal cumulus-fimbria interaction)[4]
- ❖ Alterations in peritoneal fluid may impact sperm, oocyte, embryo or fallopian tube function[5]
- ❖ Altered hormonal and cell-mediated function
  - IgG and IgA autoantibodies and lymphocytes may alter endometrial receptivity and implantation
  - Autoantibodies to endometrial antigens can be increased[5]
- ❖ Endocrine and ovulatory abnormalities
  - Endometriosis patients may have risk of the following[6]
    - Luteinized unruptured follicle syndrome
    - Luteal phase defect
    - Abnormal follicle growth
    - Premature LH surges
    - Impaired implantation

- Decreased B integrin expression (a cell adhesion molecule) during implantation[7]
- Very low levels of enzyme involved in the synthesis of endometrial ligand for L-section (a protein coating trophoblast on blastocyst surface) [8,9]

⊃ APPROACH TO A PATIENT

Initially a detailed infertility workup is completed and cause if any should be ascertained. If mild endometriosis is suspected then the patient should be treated like unexplained infertility; 3 cycles of COH with IUI. If no success then the choices are laparoscopy to see and treat if endometriosis present or to directly go for assisted reproduction. The decision would be based on factors like age, ovarian reserve, other associated factors like presence of male factor infertility or tubal disease and the financial condition.

If severe disease is present as suggested by previous laparoscopic surgery or clinical picture or imaging modalities like ultrasound and MRI, then directly proceeding to IVF-ICSI would be the prudent choice. Other indications for directly proceeding to IVF are age> 35 years, semen abnormality, poor tubal condition or poor ovarian reserve. Failure to conceive within 12 months of surgery is also an indication for IVF. **(Flow chart 5.1)**

Flow chart 5.1: Management of infertility associated with endometriosis

* AMH- Anti Mullerian Hormone
** AFH- Antral Follicular Count

⊃ MEDICAL MANAGEMENT

Medical management of infertility related to endometriosis in the form of hormonal suppression is ineffective and should not be offered as first line of management.[10]

⊃ SURGICAL MANAGEMENT

Surgery is preferably performed by laparoscopy as it seems less adhesiogenic and requires shorter hospital stay compared to laprotomy.[11]

The issue of whether surgery improves the chances of a women conceiving spontaneously (naturally) is complex.

But both the Cochrane reviews and the RCOG guidelines are in agreement that there is definite improvement in fertility associated with endometriosis following laparoscopic surgery.[12] Ablation of endometriotic implants as well as adhesiolysis to improve fertility is more effective than just diagnostic laparoscopy alone. In addition, pain relief is an added advantage.

However, only 1 additional pregnancy will occur among every 8 patients undergoing laparoscopy.[12]

For ovarian endometriomas, the green top guidelines clearly state that laparoscopic cystectomy is better than drainage and coagulation.[13] The Cochrane review suggests that cystectomy is associated with lesser recurrences of endometriomas as well as recurrence of pain than drainage and coagulation. Excisional surgeries also provide the benefit of providing tissue for histology but there is a risk of loss of healthy ovarian tissue and decrease in ovarian reserve. Randomized controlled trials showed that the excision technique is associated with a higher pregnancy rate and a lower rate of recurrence although it may determine severe injury to the ovarian reserve.[14,15] Improvements to this latter aspect may be represented by a combined excisional-vaporization technique or by replacing diathermy coagulation with surgical ovarian suture. Barrier agents reduce but not eliminate the postsurgical adhesion formation in women with endometriosis. Encouraging evidence has been reported with interceed, Oxiplex/AP gel and Adept solution. However, available studies are mainly based on II look laparoscopies performed few weeks after the intervention and data on fertility is lacking. Clinical trials including pregnancy rate as a specific outcome are warranted.

Clinical Tips

* Adherence to principles of microsurgery such as diligent hemostasis, reduced fulguration, and limited use of sutures may improve fertility
* Excision is preferred over fenestration, drainage, or ablation of the cyst lining for the treatment of an ovarian endometrioma
* Use of adhesion-prevention adjuncts may help reduce adhesion formation but improvement in fertility is unknown.

⊃ ROLE OF SURGERY BEFORE IVF

Commonly in clinical practise it is found that endometriomas are present in many patients who are planning to undergo IVF.

Surgical excision always carries the risk of reducing the ovarian reserve by reducing the amount of healthy tissue remaining. But non removal of endometriomas might have certain drawbacks such as increasing the risk of infection, rupture and follicular fluid contamination during oocyte retrieval. Both the ESHRE and RCOG have recommended surgical excision when an endometrioma has a diameter more than 3 cm as probably size more than this may cause difficulties during oocyte pickup. Whereas ASRM does not give a recommendation, but emphasizes that the benefit of such a procedure is doubtful.[16]

Surgery before IVF is also needed if there is hydrosalphinx .If salpingectomy is surgically challenging due to the extent of endometriotic disease, then either proximal resection, clipping or even aspiration at time of IVF can be the options.

⊃ ASSISTED REPRODUCTION

Controlled Ovarian Stimulation and IUI

There is evidence from several RCT that controlled ovarian stimulation combined with IUI may be effective in improving fertility in patients with endometriosis.

IVF

If a patient with known endometriosis is to undergo IVF, GnRH agonist suppression with HT adds back for 3 to 6 months before IVF is associated with an improved pregnancy rate.[17]

Gonadotropin releasing hormone agonists (GnRH-a) in ovarian stimulation protocols are used to prevent possible deleterious effects of premature LH surges in ART. The IVF-embryo transfer outcomes after a long protocol with GnRH-a and stimulation with hMG/hCH in patients with stage I–II endometriosis demonstrate similar outcomes of IVF-embryo transfer as in those of the patients with tubal infertility.[18]

GnRH antagonist could act as a reasonable choice for poor responder patients in IVF cycles as they cause immediate suppression of LH. The use of GnRH antagonist may be rational for IVF cycles in patients with decreased ovarian reserve due to ovarian endometrioma and after its surgical treatment.

ESHRE guidelines recommend that IVF treatment is suitable for endometriosis-associated infertility, particularly for cases involving impaired tubal function, male factor infertility, and/or failure of other treatments (recommendation grade B, evidence level 2b). Moreover, endometriosis is associated with lower IVF pregnancy rates than tubal infertility (recommendation grade A, evidence level 1a).

Finally, prolonged GnRHa treatment prior to IVF should be considered for cases of moderate–severe endometriosis, as it has been associated with increased pregnancy rates (recommendation grade A, evidence level 1b)

Indications for IVF
Age ≥ 35
↓ Ovarian reserve
Severe endometriosis
Failure to conceive after surgery > 12 M
Associated tubal / male factor infertility

Clinical Tips

❖ Three months of suppression with a GnRH agonist and HT addback before IVF in women who have pelvic pain and infertility associated with endometriosis will greatly improve quality of life and reduce discomfort during ovarian

❖ Stimulation and oocyte retrieval

❖ Women with endometriosis-related infertility over the age of 35 years should be referred for IVF.

➲ REFERENCES

1. Nothnicle WB. Novel targets for the treatment of endometriosis expert opinion the targets. 2004;8(5);459-71.
2. The Practice Committee of the American Society for Reproductive Medicine. Endometriosis and infertility. Fertil Steril. 2004;81:1441–6.
3. Holoch Kristin J, Lessey Bruce A. Clinical Obstetrics and Gynecology. 2010;53(2): 429-38.
4. Schenken R S, Asch R H, Williams R F, Hodgen G D. Etiology of Infertility in monkeys with endometriosis: Luteinized unruptured follicles, luteal phase defects, pelvic adhesions, and spontaneous abortions. Fertil Steril. 1984;41:122-30.
5. Suginami H, Yano K. An ovum capture inhibitor (OCI) in endometriosis peritoneal fluid: An OCI-related membrane responsible for fimbrial failure of ovum capture. Fertil Steril. 1988;50: 648-53.
6. Lebovic DI, Mueller MD, Taylor RN. Immunobiology of endometriosis. Fertil Steril 2001;75:1-10.
7. Lessey BA, Castelbaum AJ, Sawin SW, Buck CA, Schinnar R, Bilker W, et al. Aberrant integrin expression in the endometrium of women with endometriosis. J Clin Endocrinol Metab 1994;79:643-9.
8. Genbacev OD, Prakobphol A, Foulk RA, Krtolica AR, Ilic D, Singer MS. Trophoblast L-selectin-mediated adhesion at the maternal fetal interface. Science 2003;299: 405-8.
9. Kao LC, Germeyer A, Tulac S, Lobo S, Yang JP, Taylor RN, et al. Expression profiling of endometrium from women with endometriosis reveals candidate genes for disease-based implantation failure and infertility. Endocrinology. 2003;144:2870–81.
10. Hughes E, Brown J, Col lins JJ, Farquhar C, Fiedorkow DM, Vandekerckhore P. Ovulation suppression for endometriosis. Cochrane Data Base Syst Rev. 2007;18(3):CD000155.

11. Winkel CA. Evaluation and management of women with endometriosis. Obstet Gynecol. 2003;102:397–408.
12. Marcoux S, Maheux R, Bérubé S. Laparoscopic surgery in infertile women with minimal or mild endometriosis. Canadian Collaborative Group on Endometriosis. N Engl J Med. 1997;337:217–22.
13. Royal College of Obstetricians and Gynaecologists. The investigation and management of endometriosis (green-top guideline; no. 24). London (England): RCOG;2006:3.
14. Exacoustos C, Zupi E, Amadio A, et al. Laparoscopic removal of endometriomas: sonographic evaluation of residual functioning ovarian tissue. Am J Obstet Gynecol. 2004;191:68.
15. Ragni G, Somigliana E, Benedetti F, et al. Damage to ovarian reserve associated with laparoscopic excision of endometriomas: A quantitative rather than a qualitative injury. Am J Obstet Gynecol. 2005;193:1908.
16. Vercellini P, Somigliana E, Vigano P, et al. Surgery for endometrios is associated infertility: A pragmatic approach. Hum Reprod. 2009;24(2):254–69.
17. Endometriosis: diagnosis and management. Society of Obstetricians and Gynecologists of Canada. JOGC 2010;32(7):S4.
18. Metal-Vrtovec H, Tomazevic T, Verdenik I. Infertility treatment by in vitro fertilization in patients with minimal or mild endometriosis. Clin Exp Obstet Gynecol 2000;27:191-3.

6

Endometriosis in Adolescent

◀ Vidya V Bhat, Shwetha Pramod

⊃ INTRODUCTION

Endometriosis is a cause of both pain and infertility in women of reproductive age. It may start at an early age and the symptoms of endometriosis may begin in adolescence. The Endometriosis Association registry reports that 38% of women with endometriosis had symptoms starting before age 15 years and that when symptoms begin before age 15, these girls saw physician on an average of 4.2% to that age group. Early diagnosis and referral will help young women receive the necessary education about their symptoms and appropriate treatment. Endometriosis occurs in adolescents as early as 8 years of age. There have been documented cases of endometriosis occurring prior to menarche.

Adolescents presenting with chronic pelvic pain are treated with cyclic combination oral contraceptive pills and nonsteroidal anti-inflammatory agents. If the pain does not respond to these therapies, or a palpable mass in felt per abdomen, then in adolescents as in adults, an operative laparoscopy is recommended for the diagnosis and surgical management of endometriosis. Adolescents tend to have clear, red, white, and/or yellow-brown lesions more frequently than black or blue lesions. Subtle clear lesions of endometriosis may be better visualized by filling the pelvis with irrigation fluid so that the clear lesions can be appreciated in a three-dimensional appearance. Young women who are found to have endometriosis by laparoscopy may present with acyclic, cyclic, and constant pelvic pain. Adolescents with pelvic pain not responding to conventional medical therapy have approximately a 70% prevalence of endometriosis. It is known that endometriosis is a progressive disease and since there is no cure, adolescents with endometriosis require long-term medical management until the time in their lives when they have completed childbearing. Psychosocial support is extremely important for this population of young women with endometriosis.

Although symptoms of pain are reported by almost one-third of all gynecological patients, and about 50% of menstruating adolescents and young women suffer from painful menstruation (OÈ zaksit, et al. 1995), endometriosis should be suspected in adolescents because it is a common cause of pain and dysmenorrhea, affecting 45±70% of those with chronic pelvic pain (Propst and Laufer, 1999). One study comparing preoperative pelvic examination and ultrasonographic endings with laparoscopy in 45 adolescents with chronic pelvic pain showed that when both, pelvic examination and ultrasound were normal, 50% of these cases were abnormal at laparoscopy and 20% of them had endometriosis (OÈ zaksit et al. 1995).

Geographic Incidence

A genetic predisposition to endometriosis has been supported by the high concordance of the disease among identical twins. A familial predisposition with no clear Mendelian inheritance, but rather with multifactorial polygenic traits, has been identified in severe endometriosis and a number of genetic polymorphisms have been investigated. Although Chatman et al reported that there is no known racial or socioeconomic bias for the disease, it has been suggested that Asian women are at higher risk than other races, with Black women at lower risk. However, this latter finding was attributed to a frequent misdiagnosis of Black women as having pelvic inflammatory disease rather than endometriosis. Menstrual and reproductive factors associated with lifestyle factors, such as smoking, exercise, and consumption of alcohol and caffeine, have been related to altered risk of endometriosis. Smoking has been found to create a hypoestrogenic state inversely related with endometriosis, but others have found no association. Increased caffeine and alcohol consumption has been associated with increased risk, whereas regular exercise reduces the risk of endometriosis.

Although Signorello et al. did not find any relationship to alcohol or smoking, they confirmed that exercising more than 4 hour per week decreases the risk of endometriosis.

Exposure to polychlorinated biphenyl (PCB) and dioxin has been associated with endometriosis in studies with rhesus monkeys, possibly through effects on the immune system. In humans, studies of toxin exposure as measured by serum levels have been contradictory. Positive associations of PCB congeners, heavy metals, chlorinated pesticides, and dioxin with endometriosis have been reported, although other studies found no association with organic pollutants, 30 or found only a nonsignificant doubling of risk with dioxin. *In utero* exposures may also determine a woman's risk of having endometriosis. Greater birthweight and breastfeeding were found to decrease endometriosis risk, while diethylstilbestrol exposure and multiple pregnancies increased the risk.

⊃ PREVALENCE

The overall incidence of adolescent endometriosis may be different to obtain. Endometriosis has been diagnosed by laparoscopy among adolescent girls and young women (under 19 to 21 years) with dysmenorrhea and chronic pelvic pain not controlled by NSAIDs or CHCs at rates between 35.5% and 70% to 73%. Which may of undiagnosed. Endometriotic-like lesions (vascular proliferation, hemosiderin deposits, stroma but no endometrial glands) have been documented in premenarcheal girls with breast sexual maturity ratings of I to III and no Müllerian anomalies. Treatment of the lesions reduced the pelvic pain. Hence, the onset of thelarche may be considered a developmental milestone at which endometriosis should be considered in the differential diagnosis of pelvic pain.

Presentation

There could be initial delay in the diagnosis endometriosis because the pain may be attributed to normal port of growing. When pelvic pain interferes with daily activities (such as school and work) it requires attention and management.

Ten percent of dysmenorrhea in adolescents is secondary to other conditions. Endometriosis is the most common cause of secondary dysmenorrhea in adolescents. As primary dysmenorrhea occurs with the establishment of ovulatory cycles (inmid- and late adolescence), the onset of dysmenorrhea soon after the onset of menarche (within the first 6 months) should raise the consideration of a secondary cause and, in particular, asymmetrically obstructed outflow tracts with Müllerian anomalies. Coexistence of endometriosis and obstructed outflow tracts is presumed to be due in part to excess retrograde menstruation. Congenital anomalies of the reproductive tract have been found in up to 11% of adolescents with endometriosis, and endometriosis is reported to be present in up to 76% of patients with Müllerian anomalies and outflow tract obstruction.[6] Initial surgery can be limited to relief of the obstruction, since this may be followed by resolution of the endometriosis. Adolescents with endometriosis have a variable pain history.

Whereas 9.4% will complain of cyclic pain alone, more than 90% have an acyclic pain pattern with or without dysmenorrhea.

⊃ DIAGNOSIS

The approach to diagnosing endometriosis in adolescents should include detailed history-taking, an age-appropriate physical examination, and diagnostic imaging. As adolescents may have limited experience with seeking health care for gynecologic issues, establishing rapport is important. A health risk screening tool such as the HEADSS assessment may assist the health care provider. HEADSS is a framework for history-taking that begins with topics the adolescent may have more comfort discussing and concludes with more sensitive questions: **H**ome or housing, **e**ducation and employment, **a**ctivities, **d**rugs, **s**exual activity and sexuality, and **s**uicide and depression. Privacy and confidentiality should be explained to both the adolescent and her family early on the health care visit.

Completing a pelvic examination of the young adolescent may be challenging; however, it is valuable to help rule out pelvic masses and obstructive outflow tract anomalies. Flexibility should be applied when deciding on the extent of an examination. Whereas patients with a completely obstructed outflow tract (e.g. with an imperforate hymen or a transverse vaginal septum) may present with cyclic pain, they also will have primary amenorrhea and often a pelvic mass. Inspection of the external genitalia, with separation and traction of the labia, may demonstrate low outflow tract anomalies. Ruling out asymmetric outflow tract anomalies such as obstructing hemivaginal septum and non-communicating functional uterine horns, which may cause severe cyclic pain, is important. It may be possible to insert a cotton-tipped swab into the vagina to ensure that it is of normal length if a bimanual and speculum examination is not possible. A rectoabdominal examination allows palpation for pelvic masses. For older, sexually active adolescents, a physical examination is important to rule out other causes of pain, such as pelvic inflammatory disease, ovarian cysts, and complications of pregnancy. The physical findings will often be normal in this age group even when endometriosis is present. A perrectal examination will help to diagnose Culdesac nodularity, adnexal masses, and a fixed, retroverted uterus are uncommon in adolescents with endometriosis, as the disease is predominantly ASRM stage I or II. Deeply infiltrating endometriosis, although uncommon, may occur in adolescents. Rectovaginal, uterovesical, full-thickness bowel, and ureteric endometriosis have been diagnosed in this age group, although at a median age of 19 years. Pelvic imaging is an adjunct for diagnosis in the adolescent. Pelvic imaging with ultrasonography and MRI is essential if a Müllerian anomaly is suspected.

➲ MANAGEMENT

Empiric treatment with NSAIDs and CHCs is appropriate for most adolescents with dysmenorrhea. However, patients who do not respond to these medications require early referral for further investigations, which may include laparoscopy for diagnosis and treatment. There is very limited information on response to either medical or surgical therapy in this age group. Although all medical and surgical options for endometriosis may be included in the care of adolescents, the health care provider needs to consider the patient's age and the side-effect profiles of the various agents; in particular, there is potential for bone loss with GnRH agonists and depot progestin. A stepwise approach is usual for medical management, starting with CHC therapy in an extended or continuous fashion. Empiric GnRH agonist therapy with HT addback is reserved for adolescents over the age of 18 years owing to the concern of detrimental effects on BMD. With confirmation of an endometriosis diagnosis at surgery, continuous therapy with a CHC or a GnRH agonist with HT addback may be prescribed for adolescents as young as 16 years who have persistent problematic pelvic pain.

A GnRH agonist is generally not recommended for patients under the age of 16 years. If GnRH agonist with HT addback therapy is prescribed, general advice about bone health maintenance, such as supplemental calcium and vitamin D intake, should be provided and consideration given to the monitoring of BMD. Anecdotal experience with an LNG-IUS has been reported. The timing of surgical management of endometriosis in adolescents is controversial. Laparoscopy, if performed, should be done by experienced surgeons who will recognize that younger patients have atypical endometriotic lesions, with more clear vesicles and red lesions and fewer classic "powder-burn" lesions, and should include resection or ablation of lesions for pain treatment. Laparoscopy can confirm endometriosis before the introduction of GnRH agonist therapy when adolescents have pervasive pelvic pain despite initial medical therapy. The literature on outcomes of surgical resection of endometriotic lesions in adolescents is limited and involves small numbers of patients. In a study of 11 surgically treated women under age 21 years who had mild, moderate, or severe endometriosis and were given postoperative medical management (LNG-IUS, extended use of CHCs, or DMPA), 8 either became completely pain-free or had greatly reduced pain. Others have demonstrated an up to 84% reduction in symptoms.

In severe endometriosis laparoscopic surgery should be performed by level III surgical ` by level III surgical skill and set up. There is risk of complications in the extensive surgery. As for as possible bowel resection and colostomy should be avoided laparotomy should be the last resort as it can lead to psychological and social problems in the adolescents.

Like other women with chronic pelvic pain, adolescents may be helped by multimodal therapy and a biopsychosocial model of care. Behavioral modification techniques (such as biofeedback, relaxation, and hypnosis), cognitive therapy, and complementary therapies (such as acupuncture) may be used in a multidisciplinary approach. Long-term medical therapy will hopefully decrease pain and the progression of the disease, thus decreasing the risk of advanced-stage disease and infertility.

➲ SUMMARY STATEMENTS

1. Endometriosis is the most common cause of secondary dysmenorrhea in adolescents (II-2).
2. Adolescents with endometriosis are more likely than adult women to present with acyclic pain (III).
3. The physical examination of adolescents with endometriosis will rarely reveal abnormalities, as most will have early-stage disease (II-2).

Clinical Tip

The approach to pelvic examination in adolescents should be flexible. Inspection, a rectoabdominal examination, and testing of the length of the vagina with a cotton-tipped swab can be used in not sexually active adolescents to investigate secondary dysmenorrhea.

Recommendations

1. Endometriosis in adolescents is often early stage and atypical. Laparo-scopists should look intra-abdominally for clear vesicles and red lesions in adolescents (II-2B).
2. All available therapies for endometriosis may be used in adolescents, but the age of the patient and the side-effect profiles of the medications should be considered (III-A).

○ BIBLIOGRAPHY

1. Al-Jefout M, Palmer J, Fraser IS. Simultaneous use of a levonorgestrel intrauterine system and an etonogestrel subdermal implant for debilitating adolescent endometriosis. Aust N Z J Obstet Gynaecol 2007;47:247–9.
2. Arruda MS, Petta CA, Abrao MS, Benette–Pinto CL. Time elapsed from onset and symptoms to diagnosis of endometriosis in a short study of Brazilian women. Hum Reprod 2003;18(4):756-9.
3. Ballweg ML. Big picture of endometriosis helps provide guidance on approach to teens: comparative historical data show endo starting younger, is more severe. J Pediatr Adolesc Gynecol 2003;16(3):S21–6.
4. Candiani GB, Fedele L, Candiani M. Double uterus, blind hemivagina, and ipsilateral renal agenesis: 36 cases and long-term follow-up. Obstet Gynecol 1997;90:26–32.
5. Davis AR, Westhoff C, O'Connell K, Gallagher N. Oral contraceptives for dysmenorrhea in adolescent girls. Obstet Gynecol 2005;106:97–104.
6. Davis GD, Thillet E, Lindemann J. Clinical characteristics of adolescent endometriosis. J Adolesc Health. 1993;14:362–8.
7. DiVasta AD, Laufer MR, Gordon C. Bone density in adolescent treated with a GnRH agonist and addback therapy for endometriosis. J Pediatr Adolesc Gynecol 2007;20:293–7.
8. Emmert C, Romann D, Riedel HH. Endometriosis diagnosed by laparoscopy in adolescent girls. Arch Gynecol Obstet. 1998;261:89–93.
9. Goldstein DP, De Cholnoky C, Emans SJ. Adolescent endometriosis. J Adolesc Health Care 1980;1:37–41.
10. Gover S. Pelvic pain in the female adolescent. Aust Fam Physician 2006;35:850–3.
11. Greco D. Management of adolescent chronic pelvic pain from endometriosis: A pain center perspective. J Pediatr Adolesc Gynecol. 2003;16(3 Suppl):S17–9.
12. Harel Z. A contemporary approach to dysmenorrhea in adolescents. Pediatr Drugs 2002;4:797–805.
13. Laufer MR, Goietein L, Bush M, Cramer DW, Emans SJ. Prevalence of endometriosis in adolescent girls with chronic pelvic pain not responding to conventional therapy. J Pediatr Adolesc Gynecol. 1997;10:199–202.
14. Laufer MR, Sanfilippo J, Rose G. Adolescent endometriosis: diagnosis ad treatment approches. J pediatr Adolesc Gynecol 2003;16(3):S3-11.
15. Marsh EE, Laufer MR. Endometriosis in premenarcheal girls who do not have an associated obstructed anomaly. Fertil Steril 2005;83:758–60.
16. Olive D, Henderson D. Endometrosis and Müllerian anomalies. Obstet Gynecol 1987;69:412–5.

17. Reese KA, Reddy S, Rock JA. Endometriosis in an adolescent population: the Emory experience. J Pediatr Adolesc Gynecol 1996;9:125–8.
18. Sanfilippo J, Wakim N, Schikler K, Yussman M. Endometriosis in association with uterine anomaly. Am J Obstet Gynecol. 1986;154:39–43.
19. Stavroulis AI, Saridogan E, Creighton SM, Cutner AS. Laparoscopic treatment of endometriosis in teenagers. Eur J Obstet Gynecol Reprod Biol. 2006;248–50.
20. Templeman C. Adolescent endometriosis. Obstet Gynecol Clin North Am 2009;36: 177–86.
21. Vercellini P, Fedele L, Arcaini L, Bianchi S, Rognoni M, Candiani G. Laparoscopy in the diagnosis of chronic pelvic pain in adolescent women. J Reprod Med. 1989;34: 827–30.
22. Wayne PM, Kerr CE, Schnyer RN, Legedza ATR, Savetsky-German J, Shields MH, et al. Japanese-style acupuncture for endometriosis-related pelvic pain in adolescents and young women: Results of a randomized sham-controlled trial. J Pediatr Adolesc Gynecol. 2008;21:247–5.

Adenomyosis an Enigma

◀ Rishma Dhillon Pai, Hrishikesh D Pai, Rutvij Dalal

Adenomyosis is the presence of endometrial tissue within the myometrium and secondary smooth muscle hypertrophy/hyperplasia. It can be diffuse or focal. Adenomyosis has often been referred to as endometriosis interna. This is incorrect because endometriosis and adenomyosis are seen in the same patient in less than 20% of women. Endometriosis and adenomyosis are most likely clinically different diseases. The only common feature is the presence of ectopic endometrial glands and stroma. Adenomyosis is derived from aberrant glands of the basalis layer of the endometrium. Therefore, these glands do not usually undergo the traditional proliferative and secretory changes that are associated with cyclic ovarian hormone production. The disease is common and may be found in up to 60% of hysterectomy specimens in women in the late reproductive years. Most studies have documented an incidence closer to 30%. Thus, the histogenesis of adenomyosis is direct extension from the endometrial lining **(Fig. 7.1)**.

The disease is associated with increased parity, uterine surgeries and traumas. The pathogenesis of adenomyosis is unknown but is theorized to be associated with disruption of the barrier between the endometrium and myometrium as an initiating step. Studies have found a higher rate of induced abortion with presumed curettage in women with adenomyosis versus controls. Many studies have noted the history of any prior uterine surgery to

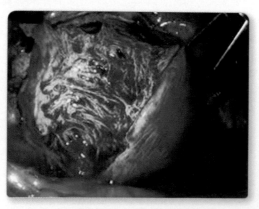

Figure 7.1: Adenomyosis

be a significant risk factor for women with adenomyosis. These studies support the theory that trauma to the endometrial-myometrial interface as a significant factor in the etiology of this condition. However, as adenomyosis may occur in nulliparous women, the full pathogenesis is yet to be determined.

➲ PATHOLOGY

There are two distinct pathologic presentations of adenomyosis. The most common is a diffuse involvement of both anterior and posterior walls of the uterus. The posterior wall is usually involved more than the anterior wall. The individual areas of adenomyosis are not encapsulated. The second presentation is a focal area or adenomyoma. This results in an asymmetrical uterus, and this special area of adenomyosis may have a pseudocapsule. Diffuse adenomyosis is found in two-thirds of cases.

In the diffuse type of adenomyosis the uterus is uniformly enlarged, usually two to three times normal size. It is often difficult to distinguish on physical examination from uterine leiomyomas. However, the ultrasound appearance of leiomyomata helps to distinguish the two. Similarly on visual inspection the two entities are quite different. When the myometrium is transected by a knife, the cut surface protrudes convexly and has a spongy appearance. The cut surface of a uterus with adenomyosis is darker than the white surface of a myoma. Sometimes there are discrete areas of adenomyosis that are not densely encapsulated and contain small, dark cystic spaces. There is not a distinct cleavage plane around focal adenomyomas as there is with uterine myomas.

On histologic examination there are benign endometrial glands and stroma within the myometrium. These glands rarely undergo the same cyclic changes as the normal uterine endometrium **(Fig. 7.2)**.

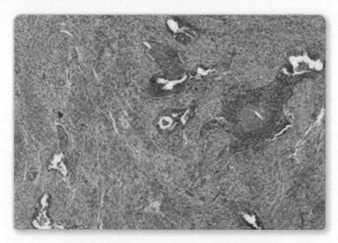

Figure 7.2: Histopathology of adenomyoma

The diagnosis of adenomyosis is made on the finding of endometrial glands and stroma more than one low-powered field (2.5 mm) from the basalis layer of the endometrium. The small areas of adenomyosis have the same general appearance as the basalis layers of the endometrium. Histologically, the glands exhibit an inactive or proliferative pattern. In general, there is a lack of inflammatory cells surrounding the fossae of adenomyosis. Although the areas do not undergo full menstrual-type changes, bleeding may occur in these ectopic areas. Some fossae of adenomyosis undergo decidual changes either during pregnancy or during estrogen–progestin therapy for endometriosis. The reaction of the myometrium to the ectopic endometrium is hyperplasia and hypertrophy of individual muscle fibers. Surrounding most foci of glands and stroma are localized areas of hyperplasia of the smooth muscle of the uterus. This change in the myometrium produces the globular enlargement of the uterus.

Symptoms

Many women with adenomyosis are asymptomatic or have minor symptoms. Symptomatic adenomyosis usually presents in women between the ages of 35 and 50. The severity of pelvic symptoms increases proportionally to the depth of penetration and the total volume of disease in the myometrium.

The classic symptoms of adenomyosis are secondary dysmenorrhea and menorrhagia. The acquired dysmenorrhea becomes increasingly more severe as the disease progresses. Occasionally, the patient complains of dyspareunia which is midline in location and deep in the pelvis. On pelvic examination the uterus is diffusely enlarged. It is unusual for the uterine enlargement associated with adenomyosis to be greater than a 14-week-size gestation unless the patient also has uterine myomas. The uterus is globular and tender immediately before and during menstruation. The association between adenomyosis and infertility is not well-defined. Destruction of the normal architecture of the myometrium leading to impairment of the uterine mechanisms for rapid and sustained directed sperm transport has been proposed as the effect of adenomyosis causing infertility.

Diagnosis

The diagnosis of adenomyosis is usually confirmed following histologic examination of the hysterectomy or excised adenomyoma specimen. Attempts have been made to establish the diagnosis preoperatively by transcervical needle biopsy of the myometrium. However, even with multiple needle biopsies, the sensitivity of the test is too low to be of practical clinical value. Adenomyosis may coexist with both endometrial hyperplasia and endometrial carcinoma. Approximately 60% of women with adenomyosis have coexistent pelvic pathology, most commonly myomas but also endometriosis or endo-metrial hyperplasia.

Transvaginal US is the initial imaging investigation, with MRI being reserved for indeterminate cases or those undergoing uterus—sparing surgery. Pitfalls in the diagnosis of uterine adenomyosis include leiomyoma, endometrial carcinoma and myometrial contractions.

Ultrasound

Transvaginal US has an accuracy of 68 to 86% in the diagnosis of diffuse adenomyosis. Typically, the uterus assumes an enlarged but globular configuration, often with anteroposterior asymmetry. Myometrial heterogeneity is related to the presence of endometrial implants and intervening smooth muscle hypertrophy. The implants present as diffuse echogenic nodules, subendometrial echogenic linear striations and nodules and 2 to 6 mm subendometrial cysts (present in 50% of cases) which represent hemorrhage within the implants. Other ultrasound features of adenomyosis include endometrial pseudowidening, poor definition of the endomyometrial junction and multiple fine areas of attenuation throughout the lesion—the 'rain shower' appearance. Color Doppler examination demonstrates a speckled pattern of increased vascularity within the heterogeneous area. While the diagnosis of diffuse adenomyosis can be suggested on transvaginal US, the findings of focal adenomyosis are hard to distinguish from leiomyoma. Because the findings may be subtle, real time or video evaluation (as opposed to static images) of women suspected of adenomyosis may be the key to making the diagnosis.

MRI

On T2-weighted MRI, adenomyosis appears as areas of low myometrial signal intensity, which presents as focal or diffuse thickening of the junction zone (JZ). When diffuse, a widened low intensity JZ >12 mm diagnoses disease with high accuracy, while a JZ < 8 mm excludes disease with high accuracy. For indeterminate cases (JZ 8–12 mm), ancillary criteria are used. These include the presence of high signal intensity linear striations (finger-like projections) extending out from endometrium into myometrium on T2-weighted images and high signal intensity foci on T1-weighted images. These foci are believed to represent endometrial rests and/or small punctate hemorrhages.

Ultrasound and MRI are useful to help differentiate between adenomyosis and uterine myomas in a young woman desiring future childbearing. Diagnosing adenomyosis by transvaginal ultrasonography has a reported sensitivity between 53% to 89% and a specificity of 50% to 89%. In some series, MRI is more sensitive, ranging between 88% and 93%, and has a higher specificity (66% to 91%) than ultrasonography in the diagnosis of adenomyosis. T2-weighted images are superior in making the diagnosis and documenting widened junctional zones. Findings of poorly defined junctional zone markings in the endometrial–myometrial interface helps confirm the diagnosis.[1] Ascher and coworkers[2] describe high signal intensity striations emanating from the endometrium and trailing into the myometrium as helpful findings. These bands most likely represent the glands and hypertrophied muscle of adenomyosis. MRI is clinically useful in differentiating adenomyosis from uterine leiomyoma.

Management

There is no satisfactory proven medical treatment for adenomyosis. Occasionally, patients with adenomyosis are treated with Gn-RH agonists, cyclic hormones, or prostaglandin synthetase inhibitors for their abnormal bleeding and pain. Hysterectomy is the definitive treatment if this therapy is appropriate for the woman's age, parity, and plans for future reproduction. Size of the uterus, degree of prolapse, and presence of associated pelvic pathology determine the choice of surgical approach **(Figs 7.3 to 7.8)**.

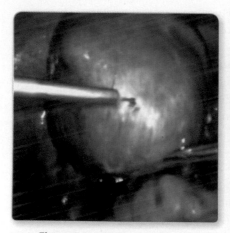

Figure 7.3: Injecting vasopressin

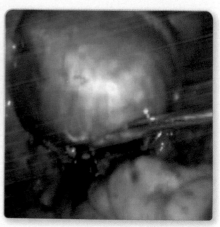

Figure 7.4: Incision on the lesion

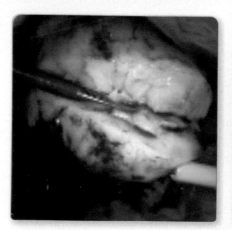

Figure 7.5: Cutting to enter the lesion

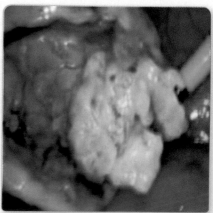

Figure 7.6: Exicision

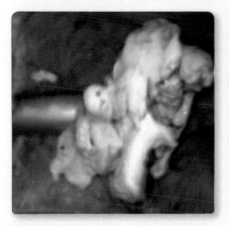 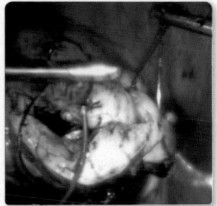

Figure 7.7: Removal of adenomyotic tissue   **Figure 7.8**: Suturing raw area

Steps of Laparoscopic Excision of Adenomyoma

Uterine adenomyosis can be focal or diffuse; focal lesions being localized in the anterior and posterior uterine walls and diffuse ones involve the entire uterus.[3] Surgical excision of focal adenomyosis have been reported in the past,[4,5] but conservative surgical treatment, rather than hysterectomy, has been reported recently for diffuse adenomyosis. Treatment of adenomyosis in subfertile patients is extremely challenging as preservation of the uterus for future childbearing is the aim and desire of all women.

To date, there is no agreement on the most appropriate therapeutic methods to manage infertile patients with adenomyosis.[6] Multiple treatment modalities including hormonal therapy with gonadotropin-releasing hormone agonists (Gn-RHa),[7] and conservative surgical procedures have been used to treat patients with unexplained infertility and adenomyosis with success.

In a study by Fathia E et al[8] the patients who fulfilled the inclusion criteria for uterine adenomyosis were allocated to 2 groups for treatment. Group A patients were treated with Gn-RHa injections alone, and group B patients underwent conservative surgery followed by Gn-RHa injections.

Conservative "cytoreductive" surgery was performed in patients with uterine adenomyosis (Group B), using a microsurgical technique.[9] The focal adenomyotic lesions were meticulously dissected and excised. The surgical margins were electrocauterized to minimize bleeding. All dead spaces were carefully obliterated with sutures. The serosa was closed with a continuous, inverting, interlocking suture of 3-0 monocryl. An adhesion barrier was applied to the sutured serosal coat. Severity of symptoms and reproductive performance of the patients were noted during the follow-up period from 6 to 36 months after all treatment was complete. Group A patients received GnRHa alone, goserelin 3.5 mg depot once a month for 6 months. All the patients in group B underwent conservative surgery followed by SC injection of 3.5 mg goserelin, every 4 weeks for 24 weeks.

In this study combined method of treatment seems to have resulted in better relief of symptoms of adenomyosis, improved pregnancy rate and a prolonged and sustained ability to achieve a pregnancy post treatment. Patients who were treated with hormones alone, seemed to benefit for a shorter period of improved reproductive performance. The combined surgical and hormonal treatment had significant benefits in giving women more effective symptom control compared with Gn-RHa alone.

The therapeutic methods of management of symptomatic uterine adenomyosis in subfertile patients is not agreed upon. The relationship between infertility and adenomyosis remains uncertain. Serial immune responses are activated in patients. Serial immune responses are activated in patients with adenomyosis causing alterations in both cellular and humoral immunity.[10] The immune changes may hamper sperm function and embryonic development that may cause infertility in patients with adenomyosis.

Currently, the accepted treatment of adenomyosis in infertile patients is with Gn-RHa. but it may be due to the transient suppression of the hypothalamic-pituitary-ovarian axis by Gn-RH agonists with resultant shrinkage of the lesions in the uterus thereby reducing its size and relief of symptoms. It probably promotes uterine and endometrial receptivity. However, its effect is often transient. Once the treatment with Gn-RHa has been stopped, recurrence of adenomyosis occurs.

The problems facing the management of adenomyosis surgically are selection of appropriate patients and the postoperative complications such as pelvic and intrauterine adhesions, future uterine deformities and reduced uterine capacity. Subsequent uterine scars may grow adenomyotic tissue and result in the reduction of its tensile strength predisposing it to uterine rupture during a pregnancy. Hence, a cautious decision needs to be undertaken in managing women with extensive adenomyosis by conservative surgery.

Preoperative diagnosis and the extent of adenomyosis with TV-USG and MRI have made it possible to select patients for treatment with conservative surgery with minimal disturbance of the uterine wall architecture. Patients most suitable for surgery are those with focal adenomyosis, where the adenoma is better to operate and excise than in patients with diffuse adenomyosis. Combination of medical and surgical methods of treatment may be appropriate in patients who do not respond to Gn-RHa treatment alone and who have severe adenomyosis causing an enlarged and firm uterus with severe symptoms of dysmenorrhea and menorrhagia. Elderly patients who do not benefit from treatment are better off having hysterectomy with conservation of the ovaries to relieve their symptoms.

No one particular method of treatment is wholly satisfactory to achieve pregnancy in the nulliparous infertile patient with adenomyosis, and patients should be made to understand this before any treatment is commenced.

Recent reports suggest that the LNG-IUS reduces bleeding and pain in women with adenomyosis and this may be a simple and effection option in women not seeking fertility.[11]

➲ REFERENCES

1. Reinhold C, Tafazoli F, Mehio A, et al. Uterine adenomyosis: Endovaginal US and MR imaging features with histopathologic correlation. Radiographics 1999;19:S147.
2. Ascher SM, Jha RC, Reinhold C. Benign myometrial conditions: leiomyomas and adenomyosis. Top Magn Reson Imaging. 2003;14:281-304.
3. Nishida M, Takano K, Arai Y, Ozone H, Ichikawa R. Conservative surgical management of diffuse uterine adenomyosis. Fertil Steril. 2010;94(2).
4. Wang CJ, Yuen LT, Chang SD, Lee CL, Soong YK. Use of laparoscopic cytoreductive surgery to treat infertile women with localized adenomyosis. Fetril Steril. 2006; 86(2):462.e5-e8.
5. Fujishita A, Masuzaki H, Khan KN, Kitajima M, Ishimaru T. Modified reduction surgery for adenomyosis. A preliminary report of the transverse H incision technique. Gynecol Obstet Invest 2004;57(3):132-8.
6. Wang PH, Yang TS, Lee WL, Chao HT, Chang SP, Yuan CC. Treatment of infertile women with adenomyosis with a conservative microsurgical technique and a gonadotropin-releasing hormone agonist. Fertil Steril. 2000;73(5):1061-2.
7. Silva PD, Perkins HE, Schauberger CW. Live birth after treatment of severe adenomyosis with a gonadotropin-releasing hormone agonist. Fertil Steril. 1994;61(1):171-2.
8. Ozaki T, Takahashi K, Okada M, Kurioka H, Miyazaki K. Live birth after conservative surgery for severe adenomyosis following magnetic resonance imaging and gonadotropin-releasing hormone agonist therapy. Int J Fertil Womens Med. 1999;44(5):260-4.
9. Wang PH, Fuh JL, Chao HT, Liu WM, Cheng MH, Chao KC. Is the surgical approach beneficial to subfertile women with symptomatic extensive adenomyosis? J Obstet Gynaecol Res. 2009;35(3):495-502.
10. Ota H, Igarashi S, Hatazawa J, Tanaka T. Is adenomyosis an immune disease? Hum Reprod Update. 1998;4(4):360-7.
11. Sheng J, Zhang WY, Zhang JP, et al. The LNG-IUS study on adenomyosis: A 3-year follow-up study on the efficacy and side effects of the use of levonorgestrel intrauterine system for the treatment of dysmenorrhea associated with adenomyosis. Contraception 2009;79:189-19.

Medical Management of Endometriosis

◀ Mandakini Parihar

➲ INTRODUCTION

Endometriosis is an important benign disease in the field of gynecology that is pathologically defined by the ectopic presence of endometrial glands and stroma within the pelvic peritoneum and other extrauterine sites and is linked to pelvic pain and infertility. It is estimated to affect 2 to 10% of women in the reproductive age group.[1-3] Although endometriosis is traditionally considered a disease of women in the reproductive age period, the natural history of this disorder, including onset and progression, has not been well-established **(Table 8.1)**.

Table 8.1: Factors affecting growth and survival of endometriotic implants

• Integrins—mainly 2B1 and 3B1
• Ultracellular adhesion molecule-1
• Vascular adhesion molecule -1
• Immune factors—cell mediated and humoral immunity
• Macrophages
• Extracellular matrix components
• Scavenger receptors
• NK cells
• Lymphocytes
• Autoimmunity
• Growth factor
• Genetic factors
• Environment factors

The hypothesis that endometriosis causes infertility continues to remain controversial. There is a higher incidence of endometriosis in infertile population than the general population; the prevalence of endometriosis in woman with infertility is about 20 to 40% compared to 2 to 10% in general female population. In some cases, the causal relationship between endometriosis and infertility is clear (as in moderate and advanced disease), but in other cases particularly with minimal and mild disease, the relationship is elusive. The incidences of endometriosis in teenagers and postmenopausal women are probably underestimated.[4,5]

Evidence based medicine allows the application of rational treatments based upon the sound understanding of the underlying pathology.

The first concept we should bear in mind is that peritoneal, ovarian and rectovaginal endometriotic lesions must be considered as three different entities. The second is to differentiate patients with minimal or mild endometriosis from those with moderate or severe endometriosis.

⊃ TREATMENT

Recently, a debate was published discussing whether the combination of laparoscopic surgery by laser, coagulation or excision and adjuvant medical therapy with Gn-RH agonists (Gn-RHa) is the most appropriate treatment for endometriosis.[29] The optimal treatment protocol is difficult to define for patients with endometriosis. We will discuss treatment options available along with an overview of the medical options available today. There is no role of medical therapy in patients with minimal or mild endometriosis. Surgical correction with sandwich therapy followed immediately by ART should be the standard of care for moderate and severe endometriosis **(Table 8.2)**.

Table 8.2: Indications of medical treatment in endometriosis

• Teenage endometriosis for pain relief
• Reproductive age group—as adjuvant to surgical correction prior to ART
• Reproductive age group for pain relief, not interested in pregnancy
• Postmenopausal endometriosis

⊃ MEDICAL THERAPY

In the last two decades, many drugs/drug combinations have been introduced in the treatment of endometriosis with varying degrees of success. These include NSAID's, combined oral contraceptives, progestogens, danazol, gestrinone, antiprogestins, Gn-RH agonists and antagonists. Disadvantages include the side effects and cost of the drugs as well as a longer duration of treatment—usually 3 to 6 months are required before there is any evidence of improvement **(Table 8.3)**.

Table 8.3: Advantages/disadvantages of medical therapy in endometriosis

Advantages	Disadvantages
1. Not operator dependant	1. Prolonged treatment
2. Less expensive	2. Side effects of drugs used
3. Avoids risks of surgery/anesthesia	3. Cost
4. Avoids risk of postoperative adhesion formation	4. Temporary relief
5. Treats lesions that are invisible to operators' eye.	

Nonsteroidal Anti-inflammatory Agent (NSAID)

Although NSAID's do not directly treat endometriosis lesions, they long have been a mainstay in the treatment of endometriosis associated pain. NSAIDS are particularly well-suited for dysmenorrhea, because the symptom is mediated by prostaglandins synthesis. By inhibiting cyclo-oxygenase, NSAID reduce prostaglandin production and alleviates pain.

Medical therapy for endometriosis can be used either as primary therapy or in conjunction with surgery preoperatively or postoperatively. This is called as the "Sandwich" therapy.

Preoperative treatment will reduce the inflammation and vascularity, thus reducing the risk of postoperative adhesion formation. It will also reduce the risk of formation of functional ovarian cysts, thus preventing unnecessary surgical manipulation of the ovaries. Usually, 3 months of drug therapy is advocated before attempting any form of surgery. The rationale behind post-operative treatment is that it will eradicate the residual implants—both visible and invisible **(Table 8.4)**. But, studies have shown that success rates are less than 30% with this form of therapy.[6] This poor efficacy of postoperative medication precludes its use in women with endometriosis and infertility as it will only further delay conception.

Table 8.4: Preoperative vs. postoperative medical therapy for endometriosis

Preoperative	Postoperative
1. Reduces inflammation	1. Treats residual implants visible/ invisible
2. Reduces vascularity	
3. Reduces postoperative adhesions formation	
4. Reduces functional ovarian cysts	

⮑ GnRH ANALOGS

GnRH analogs act by down regulating the pituitary gland resulting in a pseudomenopausal state. Today, this forms the backbone of medical therapy of endometriosis. Various doses and formulations are in use, but long acting implants produce the best results in terms of pituitary desensitization, laparoscopic scoring and histological regression.[7] GnRHa are usually used pre-operatively **(Table 8.5)**.

Table 8.5: Advantages of presurgical GnRHa treatment

1.	Reduction in pelvic vascularity and inflammation
2.	Reduction in size and activity of endometriotic implants
3.	Reduction in ovarian cyst diameter
4.	Thinning of cyst wall
5.	Absence of follicles/corpus luteum

One study, comparing the effects of leuprolide and buserelin, found that though the therapeutic efficacy of both these drugs are similar.[8] When goserelin was compared with naferelin for the treatment of endometriosis, no statistically significant difference was found in treatment results or side effects. Pregnancy rates reported after GnRHa therapy have varied between 24 to 62%.[9,10]

Side effects with these drugs are consistent with the hypoestrogenic state and include hot flashes, breast atrophy, dry skin, mood swings, decreased libido, etc. The most important of these is the trabecular bone loss 6 to 7% if used continuously for more than 6 months. This bone loss can be controlled to some extent by the use of estrogen progesterone add back therapy. This is the "addback" therapy, and is not only effective but is associated with fewer side effects.[11]

➲ COMBINED ORAL CONTRACEPTIVES

Till a few years ago, combined oral contraceptives were advocated in the treatment of endometriosis. This was mainly to reduce the frequent prolonged bleeding that is commonly associated with it. But, in view of further delaying fertility therapy, oral contraceptives are not recommended in infertile women with endometriosis. However, extensive studies have proved that COC pills are the only effective prophylaxis against endometriosis.[12]

➲ PROGESTOGENS

Progesterone acts by causing decidualization and atrophy of the estrogen dependant endometriotic foci. The action not only depends upon the dose and duration of therapy, but also upon the activity of the individual agent. Common progestogens used include medroxy progesterone acetate, norethisterone, and dydrogesterone. Depot medroxy progesterone acetate has been used as a cost effective, readily available medication with upto 66% complete resolution of endometriosis.[13,14] Side effects include irregular, bleeding, weight gain, fluid retention, breast tenderness, mood changes, depression, headache, etc.

➲ PROGESTERONE RECEPTOR ANTAGONISTS

A newly created synthetic progesterone receptor antagonist ZK 230211 has been described as having exclusive antiprogestogenic activity with minimal or no other endocrinological effects. This could prove to be useful in the treatment of endometriosis in the future.[14]

➲ DANAZOL

Danazol, a derivative of 17 ethinyl testosterone, was for the last few decades, considered to be the standard treatment for endometriosis. This acts directly on the intracellular steroid receptors, inhibits ovarian steroidogensis and also reduces the GnRH pulse frequency as well as secretion of gonadotrophins. The cumulative effects are antiestrogenic, antiprogestogenic and androgenic. It also has an immunosuppressive effect, though the importance of this action in the treatment of endometriosis is not yet established.[15,16]

As the half life of danazol is approximately 4.5 hours, ideally the drug should be administered at least every 8 hours. A minimum starting dose of 400 mg/day is adequate for most women. This is increased if necessary to suppress ovulation and relieve symptoms.[15,16] Large retrospective studies on the efficacy of danazol have reported crude pregnancy rates between 28 to 47%, with monthly fecundity rates between 4% and 6%.[17,18]

Side effects are androgenic (weight gain, acne, oily skin, hirsuitism) and hypoestrogenic (hot flashes, decreased libido, breast atrophy, depression). Another important adverse action is its effect on the lipid profile. It is no longer used in medical management of endometriosis.

⮕ GESTRINONE

Gestrinone is a 19 nor-steroid derivative with androgenic, progestogenic and antiestrogenic actions. Because of its long half life, this drug can be administered twice a week. Usually 1.25 – 2.5 mg biweekly is the recommended dose.[19] The side effects are similar to danazol, though hypoestrogenic effects are less severe. There was also a significant reduction in other symptoms such as dysmenorrhea, and pelvic pain.

⮕ INTERFERONS

The association between suppression of the immune system and endometriosis has been recently established. As a result of this, interferon therapy for endometriosis has come into vogue. Studies conducted using interferon in combination with Gn-RHa have resulted in higher cumulative pregnancy rates and monthly fecundity rates.[10]

⮕ CONCLUSION

Endometriosis is an important benign gynecology disease that is pathologically defined by the ectopic presence of endometerial glands and stroma and is clinically associated with pelvic pain and infertility. The development and growth of endometriotic lesions are estrogen dependent.

Endometriosis is the cause of pelvic pain (dysmenorrhea, dyspareunia) and infertility in more than 35% of women of reproductive age. Complete resolution of endometriosis is not yet possible but therapy has essentially main objective to increase the possibility of pregnancy and pain relief. The mean pregnancy rate of 50% reported in the literature following surgery provides scientific proof that operative treatment should first be undertaken to give our patients the best chance of conceiving naturally.

Keywords

- Pelvic pain
- Endometriosis
- Medical management.

⮑ REFERENCES

1. Houston DE, Noller K, Melton LJ. Selwyn BJ. The epidemiology of pelvic endometriosis. Clin Obstet Gynecol. 1988;31:787-800.
2. Kjerulff KH, Erickson BA, Langenberg PW. Chronic gynaecological conditions reported by US women: findings from the National Health Information Survey, 1984 to 1992. Am J Public Health. 1996; 86:195-9.
3. Punnonen R, Klemi P, Nikkanen V. Postmenopausal endometriosis. Eur J Obstet Gynecol Reprod Biol. 1980;11:195-200.
4. Chatman DL, Ward AB. Endometriosis in adolescents. J Reprod Med. 1982;27:156-60.
5. Donnez J, Chantraine F, Nisolle M. The efficacy of medical and surgical treatment of endometriosis-associated infertility: arguments in favour of a medico-surgical approach. Hum Reprod Update. 2002;8(1): 89-94.
6. Donnez J, Lemaire-Rubbers M, Karaman Y, Nisolle-Pochet M, Casanas-Roux F. Combined (hormonal and microsurgical) therapy in infertile women with endometriosis. Fertil Steril. 2007;48:239-42.
7. Donnez JA, Nisolle Pochet M, et al. Administration of nasal buserelin implant for endometriosis. Fertil.Steril. 2009;52:27.
8. Takeuchi H, et al. A prospective randomized study comparing endocrinological and clinical effects of 2 types of GnRH agonists in cases of uterine leiomyomas or endometriosis. J Obstet Gynecol. 2000;26(5):325-31.
9. Bergqvist A. A comparative study of the acceptability and effects of goserelin and naferelin on endometriosis. Gynecol Endocrinol. 2000;14(6):425-32.
10. Fedele L, et al. Buserelin vs danazol in the treatment of endometriosis associated infertility. Am J OG 1989;61:871-6.
11. Fedele L, et al. Buserelin vs expectant associated management associated with mild/minimal endometriosis. A randomized clinical trial. Am J OG. 2002;160:1340-5.
12. Tahara M, et al. Treatment of endometriosis with a decreasing dosage of a gonadotropin releasing hormone agonist (Nafarelin): A pilot study with low dose agonist therapy (draw back therapy). Fertil Steril. 2000;73(4):799-804.
13. Vessey MP, Villard Mackintosh L, et al. Epidemiology of endometriosis in women attending family planning clinics. B M J 2003;306:182.
14. Arowojulu AO. Treatment of endometriosis with depo medroxy progesterone acetate: A preliminary experience. Afr J Med Sci. 2000;29(1):55-8.
15. Fohrmann V, et al. Synthesis and biological activity of a novel, highly potent P receptor antagonist. J Med Chem. 2000;43(26):5010-6.
16. Greenblatt RB, Dmowski WP, et al. Clinical studies with an antigonadotropin danazol. Fertil Steril 1971;22:102.
17. Hill JA, Barbieri RL, et al. Immunosuppressive effects of danazol *in vitro*. Fertil Steril 1987;48:414.
18. Wingfield M, Healy DL. Endometriosis: Medical therapy. Baillieres Clinical Obstet Gynecol 1993;7:183.
19. Hornstein MD, Gleason RE, et al. Randomized double blind prospective trial of 2 doses of gestrinone in the treatment of endometriosis. Fertil Steril. 1999;53:237.

GnRH Agonists in Endometriosis

❮ Kanthi Bansal

⮫ INTRODUCTION

Agonistic analogs of GnRH have emerged as effective drugs in the treatment of pelvic pain associated with endometriosis. Iatrogenic hypoestrogenism is the fundamental mechanism through which GnRH agonists induce regression of the exquisitely estrogen-dependent endometriotic lesions. The decrease in bone mass consistently observed in women on long-term GnRH agonist treatment has prompted regulatory agencies such as the FDA to approve the use of these drugs for a maximum of six months in the treatment of endometriosis. The very high recurrence rate of pelvic symptomatology after the interruption of medical therapy underlines the importance of strategies aiming at improving the safety of effective long-term treatments. Addback regimens including estrogen preparations have been therefore studied with variable results. In strict analogy, as oral progestins have been shown to improve bone mass in postmenopausal women, regimens employing progestin addback have been proposed.[1]

⮫ GnRH AGONISTS AS A TREATMENT FOR ENDOMETRIOSIS

GnRH agonists are artificial hormones that mimic the body's natural hormone gonadotropin releasing hormone (GnRH). A GnRH agonist first leads to a rapid increase in the production of the hormones FSH and LH. However, after this brief increase, the pituitary gland stops producing the hormones, preventing ovulation.

It has been postulated that gonadotropin-releasing hormone (GnRH) analogues may act directly on endometrial cells and inhibit their growth and proliferation by regulation of apoptotic and angiogenic mechanisms. Eutopic endometrial cells from patients with endometriosis show an increased proliferation rate and are less susceptible to cell death by apoptosis than those from subjects without the disease. Notably, the GnRH analogue, leuprorelin, inhibits cell proliferation and increases the apoptotic rate in eutopic endometrial cell cultures, an effect that appears to be mediated by an increase in the expression of the proapoptotic proteins Bax and FasL and a decrease in the expression of the antiapoptotic protein Bcl-2. Angiogenesis is an important process in the development of endometrial tissue, and it is regulated by vascular endothelial growth factors (VEGFs) and angiopoietins. VEGF levels are elevated in peritoneal fluid and endometriotic tissue from patients with endometriosis. In addition, it has been demonstrated that the expression of VEGF is potentiated by a variety of cytokines, including IL-1β. Recent studies show that leuprorelin reduces the production of VEGF-A and IL-1β in eutopic endometrial cell cultures, suggesting a mechanism by which it could inhibit the development of endometriosis. Thus, GnRH analogues appear to be effective in reducing the growth of endometrial cells, not only due to their classical pituitary endocrine effects, but also via a direct effect on the endometrial cells themselves.

Mechanism of Action

GnRH agonists have the same effect on gonadotropin release after binding the type I receptor as native GnRH. The main difference of GnRH agonists used in clinical practice, in comparison with native GnRH, is that the half-life time and the bioavailability are prolonged, due to increased lipophilicity. The extensive development of GnRH agonists over the past three decades resulted in seven analogues, which have become approved for clinical use. The potency was increased by the replacement of glycine at position 6 by D-amino acids and the replacement Gly-NH$_2$ at the C-terminus by NH$_2$-ethylamide binding to the proline at position 9,[2] resulting in nonapeptides. The continuous administration of GnRH agonists (daily or depot application) initially causes LH and FSH hypersecretion (flare-up), which is followed after a period of about 10 days by desensitization of the pituitary and profound suppression of LH and FSH. This results in the inhibition of ovarian steroidogenesis and follicular growth. This "medical hypophysectomy" has shown to be beneficial in reproductive steroid-dependent disorders and during IVF treatment to prevent a premature LH surge **(Figs 9.1A and B)**.

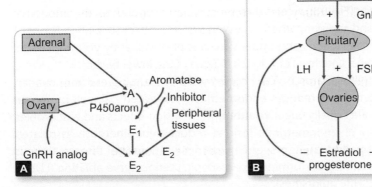

Figures 9.1A and B: A simple diagrammatic representation of the origins, target organs and feedback mechanisms of the principal hormones involved in the hypothalamic-pituitary-ovarian axis

All the GnRH agonists work in exactly the same way. When used continuously for periods of longer than 2 weeks, they stop the production of estrogen by a series of mechanisms. This deprives the endometrial implants of oestrogen, causing them to become inactive and degenerate.

Most women will stop bleeding within 2 months of starting treatment. However, some will experience 3 to 5 days of vaginal bleeding or spotting about 10 to 14 days after beginning treatment.

The return of ovulation and menstruation is very variable. Most women will menstruate within 4 to 6 weeks of their last spray of buserelin or nafarelin, or within 6 to 10 weeks of their last injection of goserelin, leuprorelin or triptorelin.

➲ DOSE AND ADMINISTRATION

At present, the usual length of treatment with a GnRH agonist is 3 to 6 months. A 3 month course of treatment may relieve pain symptoms as effectively as a 6 month course but treatment for 6 months appears to lead to a longer delay before the return of symptoms.[3,4]

The mode of administration and dosage varies according to the drug being used, as shown in the **Table 9.1**.

➲ EFFECTIVENESS

All the GnRH agonists work in the same way, so they are equally effective in regressing endometrial implants and reducing pelvic pain symptoms.[5] They appear to be at least as effective as progestins in relieving pain.[6]

For Pain

The sensory nerve supply to the pelvis can differ in amount between different women. This is most commonly believed to be the reason why some women have incapacitating pain with minimal endometriosis (lots of nerve endings in the areas of endometriosis) while other women have no pain at all despite massive endometriosis (few nerve endings in the areas of endometriosis).

Pelvic organs **(Fig. 9.2)** receive their sensory nerve supply from the autonomic (sympathetic and parasympathetic) nervous system. The sensory innervations of the fallopian tubes, uterus and upper vagina is predominantly via sympathetic fibers at the spinal cord level of T-10 to L-1 (area of the lower back).

In women with laparoscopically confirmed disease, suppression of ovarian function for 6 months reduces endometriosis-associated pain; all hormonal drugs studied are equally effective although their side-effects and cost profiles differ. Ablation of endometriotic lesions reduces endometriosis-associated pain and the smallest effect is seen in patients with minimal disease; there is no evidence that also performing laparoscopic uterine nerve ablation (LUNA) is necessary (ESHRE guidelines).

At present, the usual length of treatment with a GnRH agonist is 3 to 6 months. However, in Germany, 12 months treatment with addback therapy

Table 9.1: The mode of administration and dosage of GnRH agonist

Generic name	Form	Dosage
Buserelin	Nasal spray	Buserelin comes in a nasal spray pump. The recommended dosage is two sprays into each nostril every 8 hours (3 times a day)
Buserelin	Daily injection	A daily injection of buserelin starts with a dosage of 200 micrograms, and increase up to a maximum of 500 micrograms. The final dose Is the minimum needed to alleviate pain symptoms
Goserelin	Monthly or three-monthly injection	Goserelin is embedded in a small biodegradable implant about the size of a grain of rice. The implant is injected under the skin in the lower half of the abdomen once a month
Leuprorelin, Leuprolide	Monthly injection	Leuprorelin comes as a monthly or, three-monthly, injection that is injected under the skin of the abdomen or arm, or sometimes into the buttock or thigh muscles
Nafarelin	Nasal spray	Nafarelin comes in a nasal spray pump. The recommended dosage is one spray of the pump into one nostril in the morning, and one spray into the other nostril in the evening every day. In a few women, the recommended dosage does not stop menstruation. If symptoms persist in these women, the dosage may be increased to one spray in both nostrils morning and night
Triptorelin	Monthly and three-monthly injection	Triptorelin comes as an injection that is injected under the skin or into the buttock muscle once a month or once every three months

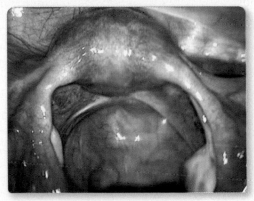

Figure 9.2: Pelvic organs

(5 mg of norethisterone per day) has been approved. A 3 months course of treatment may relieve pain symptoms as effectively as a 6 months course, but treatment for 6 months appears to lead to a longer delay before the return of symptoms. GnRH agonists are effective in relieving symptoms in 80 to 90%

of patients and the best affect is in small areas of endometriosis. Although ovarian endometriomas will shrink down by around 20%, surgery remains the optimum treatment for the more severe disease.

GnRH Addback therapy effectively treats endometriosis-associated pain, while preventing vasomotor symptoms and bone loss. It involves taking one of the following medications at the same time as a GnRH agonist: a low-dose estrogen, a low-dose progestin, or tibolone alone. The dosages used are small, so they do not reduce the effectiveness of the GnRH agonist.

Addback can be achieved by tibolone 2.5 mg/day,[7] or by an estrogen/progestagen combination, i.e. conjugated estrogens 0.625 mg combined with medroxyprogesterone acetate 2.5 mg[8] or with norethindrone acetate 5 mg,[9] estradiol 2 mg and norethisterone acetate 1 mg.[10]

Use before Surgery

GnRH agonists should not be used before surgery to reduce the extent of peritoneal (superficial implants) disease. Reducing the number and size of implants can make surgery more difficult by making it harder for the surgeon to see where the disease is present.

Treatment with a GnRH agonist before surgery may reduce the likelihood of ovarian endometriomas recurring, but the evidence is controversial.

Use after Surgery

Six months of GnRH agonist therapy immediately following surgery reduces the rate of symptom recurrence,[11] and increases the length of time before symptoms recur. It is also more effective in managing endometriosis-related pain after surgery than using oral contraceptives in the same way[12]. The benefits may be particularly relevant for women with active peritoneal disease.

Use in Recurrent Endometriosis

When used for recurrent endometriosis, thinning of the bones may be less marked during a second course of treatment compared with the first.

Role of Surgery Versus GnRH Agonist

Laproscopic surgery with cystectomy and stripping of cyst wall is treatment of choice for endometriomas > 3 cm as they respond poorly to medical therapy .In addition, hormonal suppression does not affect the adhesions often associated with large lesions.

Role of GnRH Agonists in IVF

In minimal-mild endometriosis, suppression of ovarian function to improve fertility is not effective, but ablation of endometriotic lesions plus adhesiolysis is effective compared to diagnostic laparoscopy alone **(Fig. 9.3)**. There is insufficient evidence available to determine whether surgical excision of

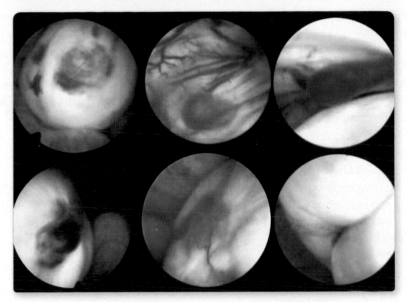

Figure 9.3: Laparoscopic view of endometriotic lesions

moderate-severe endometriosis enhances pregnancy rates. IVF with ultra long or long protocol is appropriate treatment especially if there are coexisting causes of infertility and/or other treatments have failed, but IVF pregnancy rates are lower in women with endometriosis than in those with tubal infertility. The management of severe/deeply infiltrating endometriosis is complex (ESHRE guidelines).

Impact of GnRH agonist on treatment on recurrence of ovarian endometriomas after conservative laparoscopic management

After surgery the cumulative rate of ultrasonographic recurrence has been reported to be 11.7% at 4 years and 18.9% at 5 years. The rate of recurrence is directly proportional to duration and follow-up.

GnRH agonist treatment for 6 months after surgery was reported to reduce endometriosis associated pain at 12 and 24 months compared to expectant management or placebo.

Recently an updated online version of ESHRE guidelines mentioned that treatment for 3 months with GnRH agonist may be as effective as 6 months in terms of pain relief.

Treatment with GnRH agonists for 6 months had a beneficial impact on ultrasonographic recurrence rate after conservative laproscopic surgery for ovarian endometriosis (Endometriosis Stage III/IV) at 24/36 months follow-up.

➲ SIDE EFFECTS

Hot flashes, mood swings, vaginal dryness, bone and joint aches, hair loss, lack of interest in sex, and possible short-term memory loss, menopause-like symptoms. In some cases, patients may not get relief from their endometriosis pain.

Menopausal-Type Symptoms

The side effects of the GnRH agonists are largely the result of the low levels of estrogen in the body, so they are usually confined to the symptoms associated with the menopause.

Side effects are common, and most women will experience at least one or two. The severity of the side effects varies from mild to severe, and some women will find them intolerable.

Most women will experience hot flushes or night sweats or both. The other common side effects are:

* Insomnia
* Decreased libido
* Headaches
* Mood swings
* Vaginal dryness
* Change in breast size
* Acne
* Muscle pains
* Dizziness
* Depression.

The menopausal-type symptoms usually disappear soon after treatment ceases.

Osteoporosis

The most serious side effect of treatment with a GnRH agonist is retreating of the bones, particularly the bones of the spine. The matrix that makes up bones is constantly breaking down and regenerating. When the levels of estrogen in the body are low, the rate of breakdown becomes greater than the rate of regeneration, so the bone matrix becomes less dense or thinner. The decrease in bone density is typically about 4 to 6% at the end of a 6 months course of treatment.

It is thought that most of the bone lost during treatment regenerates within 6 months of completing treatment, and that 18 to 24 months after completing treatment probably most, if not all, the lost bone has been replaced. Therefore, a single 6 months course of treatment will not usually be detrimental for women with normal bone density. However, in women at risk of developing the condition, treatment with a GnRH agonist could predispose them to developing osteoporosis.

Osteoporosis is a serious condition that can severely affect quality of life. In its more severe form, the bones, especially the bones of the spine and hips, break spontaneously. In its less severe form, the bones may just be more prone to breaking. The most important risk factor for osteoporosis is a history of the disease in a close relative, such as a grandmother or mother.

➲ CONCLUSION

GnRH resulted to maneuver the physical problems stirring due to endometriosis. The choice of symptoms and methodology of study of symptom response during treatment is very important. Since it is known that other causes of pelvic pain are also estrogen-responsive (such as fibroids or adenomyosis), improvement of symptoms during therapy cannot be ascribed with absolute certainty to improvement of symptoms caused by endometriosis. Improvement of symptoms is therefore based on the assumption that symptoms were all due to endometriosis. While endometriosis is a potent cause of pain, and while it may be true that much of the pain relief experienced during treatment may truly have been caused by endometriosis, it is not known for certain that the observed improvement represented a favorable response of symptoms due to endometriosis. Biopsy-proven evidence of persistence or recurrence of endometriosis after medical or surgical treatment, is the probable measurement which is absolutely indicative of the true response of the disease to treatment. Anything else may be a matter of opinion and not fact.

➲ REFERENCES

1. Semin Reprod Endocrinol. 1997;15(3):273-84.
2. Karten MJ, Rivier JE. Gonadotropin-releasing hormone analog design structure-function studies toward the development of agonists and antagonists: rationale and perspective. Endocr Rev 1986;7:44-66.
3. Hornstein MD, Yuzpe AA, Burry KA, et al. Prospective randomised double-blind trial of 3 versus 6 months of nafarelin therapy for endometriosis associated pelvic pain. Fertil Steril 1995;63:955-62.
4. Kampe D, Sahl AC, Schweppe K-W. Prä-und postoperative endometriosetherapie mit GnRH-agonisten in depotform: drei- versus sechsmonatige Behandlungsdauer. Zentralbl Gynäkol. 2003;125:304.
5. Schweppe K-W, Hummelshoj L. Recommendations on the use of GnRH in the management of endometriosis. In: Lunenfeld B (ed). GnRH analogs in Human reproduction. United Kingdom: Francis & Taylor. 2005:53-66.
6. Prentice A, Deary AJ, Bland E. Progestagens and anti-progestagens for pain associated with endometriosis. In: The Cochrane Library, Issue 3. Chichester: John Wiley & Sons Ltd, 2003.
7. Taskin O, Yalcinoglu AI, Kucuk S, Uryan I, Buhur A, Burak F. Effectiveness of tibolone on hypoestrogenic symptoms induced by goserelin treatment in patients with endometriosis. Fertil Steril. 1997;67:40-5.
8. Friedman AJ, Hornstein MD. Gonadotropin-releasing hormone agonist plus estrogen-progestin "add-back" therapy for endometriosis-related pelvic pain. Fertil Steril. 1993;60:236-41.
9. Hornstein MD, Surrey ES, Weisberg GW, Casino LA. Leuprolide acetate depot and hormonal add-back in endometriosis: a 12-month study. Lupron Add-Back Study Group. Obstet Gynecol. 1998;91:16-24.

10. Franke HR, van de Weijer PH, Pennings TM, van der Mooren MJ. Gonadotropin-releasing hormone agonist plus "add-back" hormone replacement therapy for treatment of endometriosis: a prospective, randomized, placebo-controlled, double-blind trial. Fertil Steril. 2000;74:534-9.
11. Hemmings R. Combined treatment of endometriosis. GnRH agonists and laparoscopic surgery. J Reprod Med. 1998;43(3):316-20.
12. Muzii L, Marana R, Caruana P, et al. Postoperative administration of monophasic combined oral contraceptives after laparoscopic treatment of ovarian endometriomas: a prospective, randomised trial. Am J Obstet Gynecol 2000;183:588-592.

Surgical Management of Endometriosis

◀ Jaideep Malhotra, Nidhi Gupta

➲ INTRODUCTION

Endometriosis is an enigmatic and debilitating disease, which occurs up to 15% of all women of reproductive age.[1]

The exact mode of development of endometriosis is unclear but it is evident that endometriosis occurs due to the dissemination of endometrium to ectopic sites and the subsequent establishment of deposits of ectopic endometrium.

Endometriosis causes dysmenorrhea, dyspareunia, chronic abdominal pain and infertility.

Various medical and surgical modalities of treatment are available for the management of endometriosis ranging from ovarian suppression with hormonal agents to radical excisional surgery. Yet, endometriosis is a challenge to the gynecologist as there is considerable confusion regarding the optimal method of management.

Treatment strategies must be tailored to the individual symptoms, age and desire for fertility. The most common approaches consist of medical treatment, laparoscopic surgery and major surgical management.

Current therapy for endometriosis has three main objectives:
1. To reduce pain
2. To increase the possibility of pregnancy
3. To delay recurrence for as long as possible.

It has been observed that endometriosis is rarely seen in the hypoestrogenic postmenopausal women which led to the concept of medical treatment by suppression of ovarian steroids and induction of a hypoestrogenic state that causes atrophy of ectopic endometrium.[2] This hypoestrogenism may also induce many unpleasant side effects. Furthermore, medical treatment has limited value in patients with infertility because it inhibits ovulation though it reduces pain in 80 to 90% of these women.[3] Medical therapy, however, is not cytoreductive and pain recurrence is frequent after treatment withdrawal.[4] Moreover, side effects and costs discourage long-term use and it has shown not to improve pregnancy rates in women with associated infertility significantly.

The actual surgical procedure performed depends on the severity of disease, size of the endometriotic cyst, availability of equipment and experience of the operator.

Advantages of laparoscopy include minimally invasive procedure and smaller incision associated with reduced postoperative pain and analgesic requirement, reduced duration of hospitalization and reduced chance of adhesion formation. The disadvantages include need for expensive equipment, operator skill, long learning curve apart from a lack of 3D perception and inability to palpate. Laparotomy may be required in "extensive disease" or involvement of rectum, ureter, etc. This again is relative and depends on the experience and skill of the operator.

For generations, it has been taught that abdominal hysterectomy and removal of both ovaries is the definitive surgery for endometriosis. However, our understanding of the disease, that it is also extrauterine has evolved and this may not be the preferred choice of treatment.

Technological advances in camera optics and electrosurgical devices, improved surgical experience, combined with the limitations of medical treatment, now make operative laparoscopy the preferred management choice for a considerable proportion of women suffering from endometriosis.

This article aims to appraise the evidence for the various surgical approaches according to the location of the disease and to discuss benefits and limitations of each and to provide to the reader the preferred choice of surgical management in different situations.

⮊ PERITONEAL DISEASE

Endometriotic implants, which are typically superficial with different appearances, can be found throughout the pelvic peritoneum.

Laparoscopic ablation with carbon dioxide (CO_2) laser was first introduced in the early 1980s. Since then other modalities have been applied, such as bipolar diathermy and techniques for excision of implants using monopolar electrosurgery, bipolar scissors and the harmonic scalpel.

Reports from uncontrolled studies suggest symptomatic relief in 60 to 70% of women following ablation of peritoneal endometriotic implants.[5]

Guildford laser laparoscopy[6] trial, in 1994, randomized 63 women with stage I–III endometriosis to either laparoscopic laser ablation or diagnostic laparoscopy alone. At the 6-month follow-up, 62.5% in the laser group were improved compared with only 22.6% in the control group. The response to surgery was poorest in those women with minimal disease. The only limitation of this trial was that, it did not permit peritoneal biopsies so it is possible that some of these women did not have endometriosis. When women with stage I disease were excluded from evaluation, the benefits of surgery improved, with 73.7% of them achieving pain relief at 6 months. In a follow-up of this cohort 12 months after surgery, symptomatic relief continued in 90% of women who had originally responded.[7]

A survey of UK practice published in 2004[8] indicated that 85% of consultants regularly perform laparoscopic surgery for endometriosis but majority use diathermy to ablate these deposits, even when there appears to be evidence for the effectiveness of laser ablation. Evidence is lacking as regards to a similar study to assess the use of diathermy, despite its popularity. The popularity of diathermy ablation probably reflects the relative availability, simplicity of the procedure and the cost effectiveness of the energy source.

According to current available evidence, it has been observed that only 62.5% of women improve following laparoscopic ablation.[6] There may be many reasons for this but one important reason for this may be that the disease may be deeper than the energy source is able to penetrate. Women with deeper peritoneal disease should, therefore, benefit from excisional surgery. It has been observed that less than 20% of consultants performing laparoscopic surgery for endometriosis use excisional methods. This probably reflects that, a higher level of training may be required to gain competency in these techniques.

Evidence for the effectiveness of excisional procedures for deeper peritoneal disease is mainly limited to retrospective case series.

A study (Abbott et al)[9] of 135 women followed-up for between 2 to 5 years following laparoscopic excision of endometriosis, demonstrated significant reductions in pelvic pain and improvement in quality of life and sexual function. However, 36% of women required further surgery for persistent or recurrent pain. Interestingly, in one-third of these women there was little or no endometriosis visible at laparoscopy.

Though, laproscopic excision of endometriosis shows very promising results in various studies, recurrence rates have also been reported. In a series of 359 women, Redwine[10] found that the maximum cumulative rate of recurrent or persistent disease was 19% achieved in the fifth postoperative year.

Abbot et al[11] trial, a placebo-controlled randomized study examining the effectiveness of laparoscopic excision for all stages of endometriosis, showed significant symptomatic improvement in 80% of women following excisional surgery compared with 32% who just had diagnostic laparoscopy. Whilst this demonstrates the benefit of surgery, the fact that 20% of women did not respond despite optimum treatment in a tertiary center should lead clinicians to continue their search for improvements in surgical techniques and advances in adjuvant therapies.

◯ OVARIAN DISEASE

Endometriomas are the endometriotic deposits within the ovary. Their pathogenesis is uncertain but are thought to result from progressive invagination of the lateral ovarian aspect after adhesion to the pelvic peritoneum. According to this theory, an endometrioma is a pseudocyst, the wall of which is the inverted gonadal cortex.

Controversy exists between two approaches to treatment for an endometrioma-excision of the cyst capsule or drainage and electrocoagulation of the cyst wall. One would expect the latter to be a superior method, if the pseudocyst theory of pathogenesis is correct. However, a Cochrane review,[12] which included two randomized controlled trials, found that laparoscopic excision of the cyst wall was associated with a lower rate of recurrence and a higher pregnancy rate when compared with drainage and ablation. The possible explanation for this could be that the depth of endometrial glandular invasion into the cortex of the ovary may be greater than the depth that most commonly used ablative modalities can reach. Despite the fact that excision of the entire cyst wall is more destructive to the ovary than coagulation, the available evidence suggests that it should be regarded as the standard and preferred method of treatment for endometriomas.

➲ PELVIC DENERVATION

Pelvic denervation can be used to interrupt the sensory nerve supply to the uterus in an attempt to reduce symptoms of dysmenorrhea. The two most commonly described and evaluated methods are laparoscopic uterine nerve ablation (LUNA) and presacral neurectomy (PSN).

Laparoscopic uterine nerve ablation involves dividing the sensory parasympathetic fibers to the cervix and the sensory sympathetic fibers to the uterus contained in the cervical division of the Lee-Frankenhauser plexus. This is achieved by creating a 1 cm deep and 2 cm wide incision in the uterosacral ligaments close to their point of attachment to the cervix, using a CO_2 laser or electrosurgery.

Presacral neurectomy involves division of the hypogastric plexus of nerves at the sacral promontory.

Comparing the two methods, LUNA can be described as a simple operation that is achievable by most laparoscopic surgeons with minimal training. PSN (because of its proximity to major vessels) has a much higher rate of morbidity and also requires much higher levels of skill and training.

Observational studies have supported the use of LUNA for primary and secondary dysmenorrhea and it has been observed that, there is either complete or substantial reduction in menstrual pain in most participants. Unfortunately, success rates have been shown to decline rapidly over time,[13] and there are concerns about anatomical distortion and subsequent uterine prolapse or bladder dysfunction by consultants.

Vercellini et al[14] conducted a randomized controlled trial comparing laparoscopic excision of endometriosis plus LUNA with laparoscopic excision of endometriosis alone. The results showed no difference in the perception of menstrual pain one year after surgery (75% in the LUNA group and 74% in the excisional surgery group).

The author's conclusion that LUNA does not give any additional benefit in terms of satisfaction or recurrence of pain for women having laparoscopic surgery for endometriosis, is supported by a recent Cochrane review.[15]

Interestingly, this review did find that PSN with conservative surgery for endometriosis was more effective than conservative surgery alone.

The largest study, by Zullo et aL,[16] reported a 'cure' rate of 86% at one year after excisional surgery with PSN compared with 57% after excisional surgery alone. Whilst these results should encourage further studies to evaluate the effectiveness of laparoscopic PSN, the complexity of the procedure with high morbidity may restrict its use in tertiary centers.

Does Hysterectomy with Bilateral Oophorectomy have a Role Today?

In conservative surgery, the endometriotic implants are excised or ablated, leaving the reproductive organs in place. Hysterectomy and removal of both ovaries is often offered as a treatment to women who have failed to respond to medical therapy or conservative surgery. Despite the lack of robust scientific evidence to support this practice, it is often described as being the definitive and preferred treatment by many consultants.

As it is defined as an extrauterine disease, it would appear irrational to remove the uterus when treating endometriosis. However, improvements in symptoms following hysterectomy and oophorectomy have been reported in many studies. This could be explained by the presence of associated pathology such as ovulation pain, adhesions, primary dysmenorrhea or adenomyosis. With this caution in mind, many studies do suggest benefits from hysterectomy if excision of extrauterine endometriosis is performed at the same time.[17]

In a follow-up study of women undergoing radical excision of rectovaginal endometriosis at Worthing Hospital,[18] those women who had a concurrent hysterectomy reported better pain scores than those in whom the uterus was conserved.

Debate remains over the benefits of concurrent oophorectomy and there are no randomized controlled trials to help resolve this issue. Results from observational studies suggest that oophorectomy has some advantages. In a series of 138 women undergoing hysterectomy for endometriosis.

Namnoum et al[19] reported that 62% of women had persistent pain when the ovaries were conserved, compared with 10% when they were removed. The relative risk for repeat surgery in women with ovarian conservation was increased by 8.1%.

Whilst oophorectomy does not appear to completely eliminate the symptoms of endometriosis, there does appear to be some benefit. Redwine[20] found that persistent pain was more common following this procedure when invasive disease was present and left in place. Fortunately, for those who remain symptomatic, excision of persistent disease can result in pain relief.[21]

Endometriosis of the Bowel and Bladder

Though, endometriosis of the bowel and bladder is considered by many clinicians to be an exceptionally rare occurrence, yet it accounts for at least 5 to 10% of cases.[22,23]

Endometriosis can involve the bowel, including the lower rectum, sigmoid colon, terminal ileum, cecum and proximal ascending colon. The depth of involvement can range from serosal to mucosal.

Bladder lesions can also extend through the wall into the mucosa and, occasionally, lesions cause such a degree of stenosis proximal to the ureteric tunnel that hydroureteronephrosis and renal destruction may result.

Medical treatment seems to be particularly ineffective in the treatment of deep disease of the cul de sac, even when combined with surgery.[24,25] Because of this, many authors have suggested the complete and radical extirpation of disease, regardless of its site.[21,22]

None of the prevalent theories of the pathogenesis of endometriosis adequately explains the site or behavior of this disease. Presence of duplication of ureters in many of these cases, may reflect a congenital abnormality of the paramesonephric duct system.

Diagnosis and staging are often difficult without laparoscopy but may be aided by transvaginal ultrasound and magnetic resonance imaging (MRI). Digital examination may identify nodules in the uterosacral ligaments or cul de sac but the detection of a nodule *per se*, even one penetrating the posterior fornix, does not necessarily imply true rectal involvement. Assessment in such cases should include an ultrasound assessment of the ureters and kidneys or intravenous urography to detect evidence of ureteric obstruction. In the presence of hydronephrosis, consideration should be given to performing a MAG 3 or DMSA scan to assess individual renal function.

Although this type of disease is usually seen during the reproductive years, it can also be seen after the menopause and even when a woman has had a hysterectomy and oophorectomy many years before. In cases where the disease first presents after the menopause there may be considerable risk of malignancy.[26]

In recent years, laparoscopic surgery has led to significant developments in the surgical management of rectovaginal disease by enhancing access to the rectovaginal space and allowing greater accuracy in delineation of disease.

Surgical techniques range from debulking of rectal lesions through disk resection to large scale bowel resections of a kind normally employed for cancer. Unfortunately, there is no current consensus as to the best approach.

In an analysis[27] of the histological findings in a series of rectal specimens removed for endometriosis, disease was present in the muscularis propria in 100% of cases. This implies that simply debulking rectovaginal endometriosis could leave significant disease behind. The same study showed that 62% of endometriotic bowel lesions are multifocal and 38% are multicentric. This would suggest that disk resection also risks leaving residual disease. Bowel resection should remove all the endometriosis but, as it is more radical, the morbidity may be higher.

Evidence suggests that radical extirpation of the disease conveys very real benefits in terms of symptom resolution and fertility, with complete or near-complete resolution of specific symptoms in upto 95% of women. Fedele et al[28] found that symptomatic disease recurrence within 3 years affected only 25% of women who received conservative (fertility sparing) treatment for rectovaginal disease. Interestingly, they found the risk of recurrence to be higher for younger women and lower if the surgery included segmental bowel resection and anastamosis. In the series published by Redwine and Wright,[29] the recurrence rate was slightly higher, with 23 women (34%) reporting the need for further treatment (13 medical and 10 surgical).

Unfortunately, there is no consistency in the surgical methods described until a properly conducted randomized controlled trial is performed. It will not be known whether complete resection with disease free margins is necessary, which method has the lowest risk of disease recurrence, or which technique has the highest morbidity in terms of rectal stenosis or fistula.

All of these surgical techniques carry a significant morbidity risk and extensive counselling is, therefore, mandatory when they are contemplated.

Surgery should ideally be performed in centers where there is a multidisciplinary team available with the necessary skills and experience to manage women with these complex issues. At a minimum, such teams must include gynecological, colorectal and urological surgeons, as well as pain specialists.

⊃ CONCLUSION

Laparoscopic ablation of endometriosis for superficial disease and excision of deep disease appear to be effective and offer significant advantages over medical therapy.

Laparoscopic surgery should, therefore, be regarded as the 'gold standard' of care. Our understanding of endometriosis, however, is far from complete and many women remain resistant to treatment. Efforts must continue to improve results further.

Efforts should also be made to preserve fertility but when this is not necessary there appear to be benefits from hysterectomy and oophorectomy, provided extrauterine disease is excised at the same time.

Whilst surgery remains the best treatment for deep rectovaginal disease, there is no consensus as to the best approach.

Evidence suggests that, laparoscopic uterine nerve ablation (LUNA) has no effect on long-term symptoms.

Developments in the surgical management of endometriosis are almost entirely the result of advances in laparoscopic surgery so that women suffering from endometriosis receive optimal treatment. We must ensure that there is adequate surgical training in laparoscopic techniques for the management of superficial disease and the organization of tertiary centers for the management of deep infiltrating disease.

➲ REFERENCES

1. Nothnicle WB. Novel targets for the treatment of endometriosis expert opinion the targets. 2004; 8(5):459-71.
2. Prentice A, Deary AJ, Goldbecle Wood, Farquhar c, Smith SK. Gonadotrophin releasing hormone analogues for pain associated with endometriosis Cochrane Database syst./J Rev. 2000;(2):CD000346.
3. Prentice A, Deary AJ, Goldbeck-Wood S, Farquhar C, Smith SK. Gonadotrophin releasing hormone analogues for pain associated with endometriosis. Cochrane Database Syst Rev 2000;2:CD000346.
4. Miller JD, Shaw RW, Casper RF, Rock JA, Thomas EJ, Dmowski WP, et al. Historical prospective cohort study of the recurrence of pain after discontinuation of treatment with danazol or a gonadotropin-releasing hormone agonist. Fertil Steril. 1998;70:293-6.
5. Davis GO. Management of endometriosis and its associated adhesions with the CO_2 laser laparoscope. Obstet Gynecol. 1986;68:422-5.
6. Sutton CJ, Ewen SP, Whitelaw N, Haines P. Prospective, randomized, double-blind, controlled trial of laser laparoscopy in the treatment of pelvic pain associated with minimal, mild and moderate endometriosis. Fertil Steril 1994;62:696-700.
7. Sutton CJ, Pooley AS, Ewen SP, Haines P. Follow-up report on a randomized controlled trial of laser laparoscopy in the treatment of pelvic pain associated with minimal to moderate endometriosis. Fertil Steril 1997 ;68:1070-4.
8. Moses SH, Clark TJ. Current practice for the laparoscopic diagnosis and treatment of endometriosis: a national questionnaire survey of consultant gynaecologists in UK. BJOG .2004 ;111 :1269-72.
9. Abbott JA, Hawe J, Clayton RD, Garry R. The effects and effectiveness of laparoscopic excision of endometriosis: a prospective study with 2-5 year follow-up. Hum Reprod 2003;18:1922-7.
10. Redwine DB. Conservative laparoscopic excision of endometriosis by sharp dissection: life table analysis of reoperation and persistent or recurrent disease. Fertil Steril 1991;56:628-34.
11. Abbott J, Hawe J, Hunter D, Holmes M, Finn P, Garry R. Laparoscopic excision of endometriosis: a randomized, placebo-controlled trial. Fertil Steril. 2004;82:878-84.
12. Hart RJ, Hickey M, Maouris P, Buckett, Garry R. Excisional surgery versus ablative surgery for ovarian endometriomata. Cochrane Database Syst Rev 2005;3: C0004992.
13. Papasakelariou C. Long-term results of laparoscopic uterosacral nerve ablation. Gynaec Endo. 1996;5:177-9.
14. Vercellini P, Aimi G, Busacca M, Apoione G, Uglietti A. Crosignani PG.Laparoscopic uterosacral ligament resection for dysmenorrhea associated with endometriosis: results of a randomized, controlled trial. Fertil Steril 2003;80:310-9.
15. Proctor ML, Latthe PM, Farquhar CM, Khan KS, Johnson NP. Surgical interruption of pelvic nerve pathways for primary and secondary dysmenorrhoea. Cochrane Database Syst Rev. 2005:CD001896.
16. Zullo F, Palomba S, Zupi E, Russo T, Morelli M, Cappiello F. et al. Effectiveness of presacral neurectomy in women with severe dysmenorrhea caused by endometriosis who were treated with laparoscopic conservative surgery: a 1-year prospective randomized double-blind controlled trial. AmJ Obstet Gynecol. 2003;189:5-10.
17. Lefebvre G, AJlaire C, Jeffrey J, Vilos G, Ameja J, Birch C, Fortier M. Clinical Practice Gynaecology Committee and Executive Committee and Council,

Society of Obstetricians and Gynaecologists of Canada. SOGC clinical guidelines. Hysterectomy. J Obstet Gynaecol can. 2002;24:37-61.

18. Ford J, English J, Miles WA, Giannopoulos T. Pain, quality of life and complications following the radical resection of rectovaginal endometriosis. BJOG.2004;111:353-6.

19. Namnoum AB, Hickman TN, Goodman SB, Gehlbach DL, Rock JA. Incidence of symptom recurrence after hysterectomy for endometriosis. Fertil Steril 1995;64: 898-902.

20. Redwine DB. Endometriosis persisting after castration: clinical characteristics and results a surgical management. Obstet Gynecol. 1994;83:405-13.

21. Clayton RO, Hawe JA, Love JC, Wilkinson N, Garry R. Recurrent pain after hysterectomy and bilateral salpingo-oophorectomy for endometriosis: evaluation of laparoscopic excision of residual endometriosis. BJOG. 1999;106:740-4.

22. Bailey HR, Ott MT, Hartendorp P. Aggressive surgical management for advanced colorectal endometriosis. Dis Colon Rectum. 1994;37:747-53.

23. Redwine DB. Laparoscopic en bloc resection for the treatment of the obliterated cul-de-sac in endometriosis. J Reprod Med. 1992;37:695-8.

24. Fedele L, Bianchi S, Zanconato G, Tozzi L, Raffaelli R. Gonadotropin releasing hormone agonist treatment for endometriosis of the rectovaginal septum. Am J Obstet Gyneco. 2000;183:1462-7.

25. Busacca M, Somigliana E. Bianchi S, De Marinis S, Calia C, Candiani M, et al. Post-operative GnRH analogue treatment after conservative surgery for symptomatic endometriosis stage III-IV: a randomized controlled trial. Hum Reprod. 2001;16: 2399-402.

26. Taylor AA, Kenney N, Edmonds S, Hole L, Notbrook M, English J. Postmenopausal endometriosis and malignant transformation of endometriosis: a case series. Gynecol Surg 2005;2:135-8.

27. Kavallaris A, Kohler C, Kuhne-Heid R, Schneider A. Histopathological extent of rectal invasion by rectovaginal endometriosis. Hum Repred 2003;18:1323-7.

28. Fedele L, Bianchi S, Zanconato G, Bettoni G, Gotsch F. Long-term follow-up after conservative surgery for rectovaginal endometriosls. Am J Obstel Gynecol 2004;190:1020-4.

29. Redwine DB, Wright JT. Laparoscopic treatment of complete obliteration of the cul-de-sac associated with endometriosis: long-term follow-up of en bloc resection. Fertil Steril. 2001;76:358-65.

Pain Management in Endometriosis

◖ PM Gopinath

The pain associated with endometriosis is the most difficult symptom to cope with for any women. It can be constant or it can be cyclical and coincide with a woman's menstrual period. In addition to pain during menstruation, the pain of endometriosis can occur at other times of the month, or for other physical or chemical reasons. There can be pain with ovulation, pain associated with adhesions, pain caused by inflammation in the pelvic cavity, pain during bowel movements, with urination, during general bodily movement i.e. exercise, pain from standing, and the final insult, pain with intercourse. But the most desperate pain is usually with menstruation and many women dread having their periods. There is also the addition of emotional pain; the emotional distress caused by this disease and the emotional pain that many people do not take a woman's endometriosis pain seriously. The pain may interfere with everyday life and may incapacitate them during the episodes in some and most of the times in many.

The problem is that it is invisible. No one can physically see what is wrong with her. On the outside she looks perfectly normal. All these things simply build layer after layer of distress and misery. This is the reality for probably millions of women around the world today. And yet most of modern society views the idea of women's pelvic pain as normal. That would be as insulting as saying that asthma is normal in children. The fact that society in general views pelvic pain as normal means that women themselves also believe that their pain is normal. This is why it takes so long for some women to realize that something is actually wrong. They may start to discuss and compare their menstrual pain with other women and gradually they realize that the amount of pain they feel is not normal.

Nearly all women with endometriosis experiences pain it in the pelvic area. The pain is often severe cramping that occurs on both sides of the pelvis, radiating to the lower back and rectal area and even down the legs. Occasionally pain may also occur in other regions. Implants can also occur in the bladder rarely and cause pain and even bleeding during urination. Endometriosis can invade the intestine and cause painful bowel movements or diarrhea. Large cysts can rupture and cause very severe pain at any time in various locations.

The severity of pain also varies widely and is not related to the extent of the disease. A woman can have very small or few implants and have severe pain, while those with extensive endometriosis may have very few signs and not suffer much pain. There is no logic as to how severe the pain of endometriosis will be, but on the whole this disease causes a lot of pain for most women.

➲ ASSESSMENT OF THE CAUSE OF PAIN IN WOMEN WITH PELVIC PAIN

Pelvic pain is assessed with a history, an examination, and special investigation.

History

Ask about the date of the last period in case of pregnancy, and make a list of each pain or symptom the patient has. For each pain, ask her to describe what it feels like, where it is, when it occurs, how many days she has it per cycle, and what aggravates or relieves it. Ask about bladder symptoms (nocturia, frequency, urine infection, urgency), ask about bowel function (constipation, diarrhea or bloating, pain opening her bowels during her period), ask about pain with movement and pain in other areas of the body (e.g. migraine or muscle tender points), ask whether intercourse is painful, and how many days a month she feels completely well.

Examination

Assess the patient's general well-being (depression, posture, and nutrition), the abdomen (for sites pain, tenderness, peritoneum, or masses), the vulva (for tenderness, skin lesions, or vulval infection), the pelvic floor muscles (for tenderness and spasm), the vagina (for nodules of endometriosis posterior to the cervix or in the rectovaginal septum, or congenital anomalies), and the pelvis (for uterine or adnexal masses, pregnancy). Vaginal examination is rarely necessary in virgins.

Investigation

Exclude pregnancy, including ectopic pregnancy, screen for sexually transmitted diseases if appropriate, and take a cervical smear if available (unnecessary for virgins). Ultrasound may show an endometriosis.

Treatment of Pelvic Pain

The treatment recommended depends on the symptoms present. Most women will have more than one pain symptom. Remember to treat any coexisting health problems to allow patient more energy to copy with their pain.

Drugs for Pain Relief

There are options available for the management of pain for women who have endometriosis. These can include a variety of drug treatments as well as natural remedies, diet changes and supplements. Drug treatment is not the best option for pain relief because of the long-term side-effects. The two pain relief drugs that are used most commonly for the pain of endometriosis are:

Nonsteroidal Anti-inflammatory Drugs (NSAIDs)

These are a class of drugs which are designed to relieve pain as well as reduce inflammation. These drugs may vary in degrees of analgesic versus anti-inflammatory activity. This means that one drug may have a great deal of anti-inflammatory but little in the way of pain reduction, whereas another drug may primarily be a painkiller with little ability to reduce inflammation. NSAID'S is a class of medications to relieve pain as well as reduce inflammation. These drugs have different degrees of analgesic versus anti-inflammatory activity where one drug may have a great deal of anti-inflammatory but little in the way of pain reduction whereas another may be primarily a painkiller with little ability to reduce inflammation. These drugs block prostaglandins, inflammatory factors strongly associated with endometriosis and increase uterine contractions that can cause cramping and pain. Be careful about using drugs that contain codeine which should not be generally used for endometriosis pain relief, they can cause pelvic congestion and constipation to exacerbate your symptoms if you have any history of gastrointestinal distress. Be advised, it takes up to 7 days for NSAID medication to become effective by reaching a steady level in the blood and up to 3 weeks to determine effectiveness in relieving your pain. There are many versions of these drugs which are available both by prescription and over the counter. Aspirin is a common NSAID; others include ibuprofen, naproxen, and ketoprofen. These drugs block the prostaglandins which are inflammatory factors strongly associated with endometriosis and which increase uterine contractions and cause cramping and pain. Drugs containing codeine should not generally be used for endometriosis pain management. They can cause pelvic congestion and constipation, which could exacerbate symptoms.

Side Effects

❖ Possible organ damage and/or addiction with extended and frequent use
❖ The most common side effects of NSAIDs are stomach upset, indigestion, and nausea.

Antiprogestins

This agents reduce both estrogen and progesterone receptors. Gestrinone is the standard agent, and may be comparable to GnRH agonists in reducing pain plus result in fewer menopausal symptoms. Mifepristone is also a antiprogestins. In a six-month study, mifepristone improved symptoms and reduced endometrial implants without causing menopausal side effects. Caution, however, this product is known as the "abortion pill" and can induce a miscarriage because its antiprogestins effects.

Effects

Gestrinone includes male hormone symptoms, to include acne, and possibly the development of high cholesterol levels.

Oral Contraceptives

Generally directed toward stabilizing the production of hormones (estrogen and progesterone) to stimulate endometrial growth. It has been found that fluctuating levels of estrogen and progestin stimulate the growth of endometriosis. Prevents the release of the egg from the ovary (ovulation). Decreases the amount of blood loss during the menstrual period. Decreases backward menstrual period flow into the fallopian tubes and out into the abdominal cavity (retrograde menstruation). Stops menstrual periods for long periods of time when taken over time. Some examples are: estrogen/progestin combination pills (birth control pills).

Side Effects

* Painful periods (dysmenorrhea) usually will return if oral contraceptives are stopped
* The risk of serious side effects is increased in menstrual periods usually are less painful with lighter flows
* Young women with very painful menstrual periods and minimal to mild endometriosis have reported improvement using a continuous 15-week birth control pill regimen program
* Continuous treatment can be used for up to 1 year.

Caution: Oral contraceptives are not recommended if one has uncontrolled high blood pressure, liver disease, history of blood clots in a vein (deep vein thrombosis) or lung (pulmonary embolus), history of stroke or if you are over the age of 35 with diabetes or if you smoke.

Danazol

Danazol is a derivative of 17-ethinyltestosterone and acts primarily by inhibiting the LH surge and steroidogenesis, and by increasing free testosterone levels. Common side effects relate to hyperandrogenism and include hirsutism, acne, and deepening of the voice. Alternate routes of danazol administration are under investigation

Gestrinone

Gestrinone (ethylnorgestrienone, R2323) is an anti-progestational steroid used in Europe for the treatment of endometriosis, but it is not currently available in the United States. The mechanism of action includes a progestational withdrawal effect at the endometrial cellular level and administered orally with doses ranging from 2.5 mg to 10 mg, administered daily to weekly. Side effect relate to both androgenic and antestrogenic effects.

Aromatase Inhibitors

In pilot studies involving very small numbers of patients, Aromatase inhibitors have been shown effective for the treatment of endometriosis, and pelvic pain. However, such treatment still is considered investigational, is not approved by the FDA for this indication, and should not be considered as definitive therapy. Endometriosis tissue, unlike disease-free endometrium, exhibits a high level of aromatase activity that may result in increased local concentrations of estrogen that may favor growth of endometriosis. At least in theory, that characteristic may help to explain observations of endometriosis in postmenopausal women and the persistence of disease symptoms in some patients receiving GnRH agonist treatment.

GnRH Agonists

The GnRH classes of drugs are becoming more widely used as means to control the pain of endometriosis. GnRH stands for gonadotropins releasing hormone. These are one of the drugs which are regularly prescribed for the actual treatment of endometriosis. They alter the natural hormone levels of the body and they chemically induce a state of menopause. This is to provide time for the endometriosis implants to shrink, as they are not being fed by the natural cycle of hormones, namely estrogen.

This method of treatment appears to be relatively effective for some women in helping to relieve the pain as well as temporarily working to shrink the disease implants. But these drugs do have many side-effects, and will affect women differently. For more information see Treatment of Endometriosis.

These drugs are only approved for use for six months of treatment. This is due to the possibility of loss of bone mass, which is supposed to be recovered after discontinuing treatment with these drugs. The option to stop bone loss during drug treatment is to give additional hormone therapy called 'Addback' therapy.

Supplements for Pain Relief

Many women have found that various natural remedies help with their pain, which are safe. These may include vitamin and mineral supplements, herbs and diet changes.

Evening Primrose oil has had good results for many women both for endometriosis and PMS. It contains a polyunsaturated fatty acid known as gamma linolenic acid, which seems to block the releases of cytokines and prostaglandins, substances that are manufactured by the endometrium and are involved in uterine muscle contraction and cramping. Foods that contain gamma linolenic acid are black currant oil and cold-water fish.

There are many changes you can make in your diet that will improve symptoms and in turn will improve the pain. This includes an array of supplements and herbs which will help to clean your system, boost your immune system, increase your energy and improve your overall health.

➲ DEPOT PROGESTIN THERAPY

DMPA, injected intramuscularly, is widely used worldwide for birth control and has been studied for the relief of endometriosis pain. A subcutaneous formulation of DMPA (150 mg), has been investigated in 2 RCTs that compared it with leuprolide acetate depot.[16,17] Over the 6-month study period, and for up to 12 months thereafter, DMPA-SC was equivalent to leuprolide acetate in relieving pain. There was some loss of BMD but not as much as in the group receiving leuprolide acetate without addback. DMPA-SC appears to be effective in relieving pelvic pain in up to three quarters of patients and is a very economical alternative in the treatment of symptomatic endometriosis.

However, prolonged delay in resumption of ovulation is a possibility, and therefore DMPA should not be suggested for women wanting a pregnancy in the near future. In addition, breakthrough bleeding may be prolonged, heavy, and difficult to correct since the progestin effect cannot be reversed quickly. Perhaps an ideal indication for DMPA is residual endometriosis after hysterectomy with or without bilateral salpingo-oophorectomy when future conception and irregular uterine bleeding are not issues. Long-term use of DMPA may be detrimental to BMD.

Immunotherapy

A variety of immune regulating medications are being considered or investigated for use in women with endometriosis. Few have yet reached the stage of clinical trials in humans; however, this will likely occur within the next few years.

One example of such a medication is pentoxifylline. Pentoxifylline is a medication most commonly used to treat patients who have problems with blood circulation. Pentoxifylline is also known to alter immune cell function. This medication has been shown to reduce the severity of endometriosis in rats and to improve egg fertilization rates in hamsters with endometriosis.

The use of pentoxifylline in women with endometriosis has been addressed in only a single study. In this study, 30 women with endometriosis and infertility were treated with pentoxifylline and another 30 were treated with placebo. After 12 months of therapy, pregnancy rates were compared between the two groups. Although there did appear to be an improvement in pregnancy rates among those women receiving pentoxifylline, the study could not prove that this was a real effect of treatment.

The use of immune therapies in the treatment of endometriosis is intriguing and may offer a more specific and tolerable alternative to the existing hormonal and surgical treatment options.

➲ TENS FOR PAIN RELIEF

Transcutaneous electrical nerve stimulation (TENS) is a drug-free method of pain relief that has been used to treat a wide variety of muscle and joint problems, as well as many other painful conditions. TENS uses electrical impulses to stimulate the nerve endings at or near the site of pain, diminishing the pain and replacing it with a tingling or massage-like sensation.

TENS can be used in a health care setting, but most often people use it at home, by purchasing their own equipment. It is a safe, noninvasive, drug-free medically proven method of pain management. There are many units available in the market.

The symptoms of pain and its psychological effects can be helped by complementary approaches.

Massage

Studies have shown that massage can alleviate muscle pain and tissue-injury pain. The considerable psychological effects of massage may also be useful for persistent pain.

Aromatherapy

Some essential oils are said to stimulate endorphin production and, when used with massage, to encourage relaxation. The stress and anxiety caused by long-term pain can cause the muscles to become tense. This may accentuate the perception of pain, creating a self-perpetuating downward spiral. So the use of aromatherapy can help to break the cycle caused by long-term pain.

Acupuncture

Acupuncture is said to work partly by stimulating the release of endorphins and prostaglandin-suppressing corticosteroid hormones. The insertion of needles in appropriate acupoints may also help relieve anxiety and depression associated with persistent pain.

Yoga and Pain Management

Yoga is believed to reduce pain by helping the brain's pain center regulate the gate-controlling mechanism located in the spinal cord and the secretion of natural painkillers in the body. Breathing exercises used in yoga can also reduce pain. Because muscles tend to relax when you exhale, lengthening the time of exhalation can help produce relaxation and reduce tension. Awareness of breathing helps to achieve calmer, slower respiration and aid in relaxation and pain management.

Yoga's inclusion of relaxation techniques and meditation can also help reduce pain. Part of the effectiveness of yoga in reducing pain is due to its focus on self-awareness. This self-awareness can have a protective effect and allow for early preventive action.

Menastil

This is quite a new product to come on the market, which is produced for the relief of menstrual cramps. Menastil is the trade name for this product, which is receiving a lot of good feedback for the relief of pain associated with endometriosis.

Menastil is topically applied (applied to the skin), using a roll-on applicator. Many women have noted how fast and effective it is at relieving their pain and cramps. It is a homeopathic preparation and is available without prescription. The active ingredient is calendula oil, which is effective as a topical analgesic and for pain relief.

Menastil works by inhibiting the pain signals as they travel from one nerve cell to another. The junction, where these nerve cells connect with each other, is called a synapse. When applied topically, at the location of the pain, menastil causes the endings of the nerve cells to retreat from each other and retract towards the cell body. This results in a reduction of the intensity of these impulses traveling to the brain and therefore a lessening in the amount of discomfort that is being registered by the brain. Quickly eliminates cramping symptoms, FDA registered, clinically proven, no known side effects, no pills to take, very affordable. Ingredients: Menastil is a blend of pure all-natural essential oils with mineral oil. The active ingredient is calendula oil, which is made by extracting the oil from marigold petals.

➲ DLPA

Endorphins are nature's pain killers. DL-Phenylalanine (DLPA) does not actually block the pain itself. It works instead by protecting the body's naturally produced pain killing endorphins (the body's morphine), effectively extending their life span in the nervous system. It slows the activity of "enzyme chewing" enzymes which destroy endorphins thereby giving them more time to act on areas of pain.

It helps the body to heal itself and working through the brain DLPA can also relieve some of the symptoms of other diseases. It is a powerful antidepressant and in clinical studies has been proven to be as effective as commonly prescribed antidepressant drugs—without the drugs' side effects. DLPA can also relieve symptoms of PMS and has had great success with deal with the pain of Endometriosis. DL-Phenylalanine (DLPA)

➲ INTENDED USES

DL-phenylalanine (DLPA) is an essential amino acid that is converted to tyrosine in the body. Tyrosine is an amino acid that is used to manufacture adrenal and thyroid hormones, and is converted into the skin pigment, melanin. DLPA was first isolated from the lupine plant.

DLPA has been shown to relieve chronic pain and to aid in the treatment of depression. DLPA works by slowing down the enzymes that degrade the biological endorphins (neurohormones) produced in the brain.

Endorphins are our "Natural" internal pain-killers and mood elevators. DLPA increases endorphin concentrations naturally and provides additional comfort against chronic (long-term) aches and pains, as well as helping to relieve depression and premenstrual syndrome (PMS) conditions.

The simultaneous consumption of small doses of available over-the-counter pain-killing drugs (i.e.-aspirin, ibuprofen, and acetaminophen) will increase the pain-relieving effects of using DLPA!

Note: DLPA must be taken on an empty stomach (1/2 hour before meal) with water (or fresh citrus juice) only for the DLPA to cross-over the blood brain barrier and be effective in relieving acute and/or chronic pain, plus depression.

Arnica Gel and Cream

Arnica is a homeopathic remedy, taken internally and used for bruises, wounds, sprains, injury, as well as for tiredness after prolonged exertion. Arnica is also used in a skin preparation for the above, and is effective for pain relief. You could experiment with both.

MSM for Pain Relief

MSM supplement for pain relief and aid healing—methyl sulphonyl methane is the full name of this natural compound. The common name for this compound is Sulfur.

MSM can help relieve pain in a variety of ways. It blocks pain messages that travel to the brain along nonmyelinated nerve fiber called C fibers. This results in relief of the deep aching pain that is characteristic of chronic conditions like endometriosis.

But MSM alleviates pain in other ways as well. It reduces the swelling and heat associated with inflammation, which in turn, relieves pressure on surrounding nerves and other tissues. It also relieves muscle spasm.

MSM goes beyond mere pain relief to actually support healing of injured tissues by increasing blood flow. It also alters the crosslinkages of collagen, reducing scar tissue to promote range of motion and flexibility.

Exercise

Probably the last thing on a woman's mind regarding help with her pain is to do exercise, but it does help. This happens because when we exercise the body produces chemicals in the brain called endorphins. Endorphins actually bring pain relief and they will surge round the body, thereby easing the pain of endometriosis. The compounds found in endorphins are of similar structure and mimic the effects of morphine, a powerful narcotic pain reliever. Ten minutes of moderate exercise is all the body needs to start producing these safe pain relievers.

For some women exercise may be too painful at times. Low impact activities may help these women. These include swimming, walking and yoga. Taking some form of exercise will help to relieve stress and tension and may reduce estrogen levels in the body. Evening primrose oil is a natural remedy which contains a polyunsaturated fatty acid known as gamma linolenic acid, that seems to block the release of cytokines and prostaglandins, substances that are produced by the endometrium and involved in uterine muscle contraction and cramping. Foods containing gamma linolenic acid are black currant oil and cold-water fish. EPO oil is an essential fatty acid used to make prostaglandins in our bodies. A theory exists that women with endometriosis may have an imbalance of prostaglandins, which are responsible for the stimulation and inhibition of smooth muscle tissue same as found in the uterus, the intestines and the bladder.

B complex vitamins have reportedly improved emotional symptoms of endometriosis and have been scientifically linked to the breakdown of estrogen in the body.

Chinese herbal teas have proclaimed to provide relief from tea made from Chinese plants and minerals. Traditional Chinese medicine identifies endometriosis as an imbalance of yin and yang, the male and female parts of the self, which can be treated by herbal remedies prescribed by a TCM practitioner.

Vitamin E and selenium are two vitamins reported to decrease endo-metriosis-related inflammation, however, medical specialists are divided as to the use of vitamin E by women with endometriosis because it boosts the production of estrogen.

Treatment of Dysmenorrhea on Day 1 to 2 of the Menstrual Cycle

Pain at this stage of the cycle is usually uterine pain. Management options at the primary care level include monophasic oral contraceptive pills, such as 20 to 30 ug ethinyl estradiol with 500 to 1,000 ug norethisterone or 150 mg levonorgestrel, as well as pain medication. The pain medication of first choice should be an NSAID taken early on in the episode of pain, such as ibuprofen at a dose of 400 mg initially and then 200 mg three times daily with food. For moderate or severe pain, opioids should be offered. Nonpharmacological options include hot or cold packs over the lower abdomen, vitex agnus catus (chasteberry) 1 g daily (avoid if pregnant; ineffective if on oral contraceptive pills), vitamin E (400 to 500 IU natural vitamin E from 2 days before period until day 3) and zinc 20 mg (as chelate) twice a day . Traditional Chinese medicine (acupuncture and herbal therapies) are also popular, but they should only be recommended if affordable and if the patient has a positive attitude.

Many women with severe dysmenorrhea become fearful as their period approaches. They fear pain that they cannot control. By providing them with strong analgesics to control severe pain if it occurs, this anticipation of pain can be reduced and they can regain control of the pain. Therefore, "on demand" doses of analgesics should be provided.

Treatment of Prolonged Dysmenorrhea

Dysmenorrhea (painful cramps) for more than 1 to 2 days is often due to endometriosis, even in teenagers. A woman with endometriosis also has a more painful uterus than other women. She thus has two causes for her pain. Managements options include on the primary care level all the treatment used for dysmenorrhea above, a levonorgestrel intrauterine device, continuous progestogen (norethisterone 5 to 10 mg daily, dydrogesterone a synthetic hormone similar to progesterone) dysmenorrhea, pelvic pain, and endometriosis.

Treatment of Ovulation Pain

Normal ovulation pain should only last for 1 day, occurs 14 days before a period, and changes sides each month. Management options include an NSAID when pain occurs, an oral contraceptive pill to prevent ovulation, or continuous norethisterone 5 to 10 mg daily to induce amenorrhea. If more than the primary care level is available, and pain is severe or always unilateral, a laparoscopy with division of adhesions and removel of endometriosis is indicated. An ovary should only be removed if severely diseased, and the patient's fertility needs have been discussed and carefully considered.

Treatment of Pelvic Pain and Bladder Symptoms

Many women with pelvic pain describe urination, nocturia, pain when voiding is delayed, suprapubic pain, and vaginal pain. Dyspareunia or the feeling of having a urinary tract infection. This feeling is often due to interstitial cystitis of the bladder. There may be a history of frequent "urinary tract infections" but with negative urine culture. First, exclude urine infection, chlamydia, and gonococcal or tuberculous urethritis. Then ensure sufficient fluid intake to avoid concentrated urine. Identify and avoid dietary triggers if present. Common triggers include coffee, cola drinks; tea (including green tea), vitamin B and C, citrus fruit, cranberries, fizzy drinks, and chocolate, alcohol, artificial sweeteners, spicy foods, or tomatoes, peppermint and chamomile tea are usually acceptable. If food triggers are present, pain usually follows within 3 hours of food intake. Provide instructions about how to manage symptom flares (drink 500 ml water mixed with 1 teaspoon of bicarbonate of soda. Take a paracetamol (acetaminophen) and an NSAID if available. Then drink 250 ml water every 20 minutes for the next few hours). For symptom control; try amitriptyline 5 to 25 mg at night, oxybutynin (start with 2.5 mg at night, increase slowly to 5 mg three times a day) or hydroxyzine, especially for those with alleries (start with 10 mg at night, increase slowly to 10 to 50 mg at night)

Many women with bladder symptoms develop secondary pelvic floor dysfunction with dyspareunia and severe muscular pelvic pain. If pain persists, consider cystoscopy with hydrodistension. All medications should be avoided in pregnancy, if possible. Also note that hydroxyzine is contraindicated in epileptics.

Treatment of Sharp and Stabbing Pains

Sharp, stabbing pains are usually a form of neuropathic pain. Treatment includes neuropathic pain medications (e.g. 100 to 1200 mg daily), regular sleep, regular exercise (start with regular low-level exercise to avoid initial worsening of pain), and stress reduction. Start all medications at a very low dose and increase slowly. Where high-level surgical skills are available, excision of endometriosis lesions, if present, can sometimes improve the pain, although frequently this type of pain continues after surgery.

Treatment of Diagnose the Cause of Dyspareunia

Dysmenorrhea (painful intercourse) may be the most distressing symptom for many women, as it interferes with the relationship they have with their husband. She may feel that she is let her husband down when she is unable to have intercourse due to pain, and he may feel that she is avoiding intercourse because she no longer loves him. It is important to identify the cause of the problem.

Examine the vulva visually for abnormalities (infection, dermatitis, lichen sclerosis):

* Use a cotton-tipped swab to test for tenderness of the posterior fourchette, even if it looks normal (to check for vulvar vestibulitis)
* Use one finger in the lower vagina to push backwards (it check for pelvic floor muscle pain or vaginismus). Use one finger to push anteriorly (to check for bladder or urethral pain)
* Use one or two finger to check for upper vagina for nodules of endo-metriosis, pelvic masses, or check for contralateral adnexal pain[9] (to check endometriosis, overian cysts, pelvic infection, or adhesions)
* Use a speculum to look for cervicitis, vaginal infection, vaginal anomaly, or endomatriotic nodules in the posterior vaginal fornix.

If any part of the examination causes pain, ask the patient if this is the same pain she has with intercourse. It is important to examine the lower vagina gently with one finger before using the speculum, or pelvic floor/ bladder pain may be missed. Generalized dyspareunia, especially where sharp pains are present, may be neuropathic. Include in the consultation a discussion about the relationship she has with her husband and whether he is supportive of her.

Treatment of Painful Vulva (Vulvodynia)

General vulval care is often helpful. The patient should not use soap and should avoid vulval products such as talc or oils. Recommend aqueous cream as a soap soother, and daily vulval moisturizer. Recommend cotton underwear and loose clothing. Treat any vaginal infection. Prescribe amitriptyline 5 to 25 mg at night or an anticonvulsant for vulval pain if present. For vulval vestibulitis, prescribe a course of oral ketoconazole (antifungal) 200 mg and betamethasone cream (0.5 mg/g) applied thinly daily for 3 weeks. For lichen sclerosis, prescribe steroid cream applied thinly daily for intermittent courses only when symptoms are present.

Treatment of Painful Pelvic Muscles

The muscles are in spasm and do not relax normally. This type of pain can be secondary to painful bladder symptoms, any type of pelvic pain, previous sexual assault, or anxiety regarding sexual intercourse. Pain is severe, just as pain from back spasms can be severe. Typical symptoms include dyspareunia (with pain for 1 to 2 days afterwards), pain on moving, pain with insertion of a finger or a speculum, and pain with tampons. There may be pain on prolonged sitting. Pelvic floor muscle spasm is involuntary, and the patient cannot "just relax". The best treatment involves pelvic floor physiotherapy, instruction in relaxation techniques, and the regular use of vaginal dilators in a relaxed, secure, nonpainful situation. Intercourse should be avoided until the problem has resolved because the problem will worsen with repeated painful intercourse. If intercourse continues, may help other treatments include:

❖ Resolution of initiating factors, e.g. bladder symptoms and pelvic pain
❖ Avoid straining with voiding or trying to stop passing urine in mid-void
❖ Regular gentle exercise (e.g. walking, stretching, gentle yoga, improved posture, sitting square in a comfortable chair with good support, keeping, and taking regular breaks
❖ Heat packs to the pelvis and a warm bath 1 to 2 times daily for 3 to 6 weeks
❖ Management of anxiety and depression, if present.

Common Barriers to Effective Pain Management

A long delay between the beginning of symptoms and management of pelvic pain is common for many reasons. The patient's family may not believe that her pain is real and severe. She may believe that severe pain with periods is normal, or her local doctor may believe that she is too young for endometriosis or underestimate how severe her pain is.

Other barriers to effective pain management include fear of gynecological examination, especially where a female doctor is unavailable; fear of surgery, infertility, and cancer; and fear of the unknown.

Dysmenorrhea, Pelvic Pain and Endometriosis

It is there important to explain to the patient and her family:

❖ The pain is real, and the pain is not her fault
❖ She does not have cancer, and her pain is not life threatening
❖ Although it may not be possible to completely cure all her pain. She can optimistically look forward it less pain and living better with what pain remains. It is important to be positive

❖ Resources she can contact if she needs help.
❖ What extra pain relief can use if the pain becomes more severe; her anxiety will decrease when she knows that she can manage pain if it occurs
❖ To ensure that she is not overworked, because tiredness will worsen her pain
❖ To ensure that she has activities in her life that she enjoys.

Points to Ponder

❖ Most women with chronic pelvic pain have several different pain symptoms. Each pain needs to be assessed, and treatment plan made. Pelvic pain cannot be considered as a single entity
❖ Many common causes of pelvic pain cannot be seen during an operation, including bladder pain, neuropathic pain, uterine pain, pelvic floor muscle pain, and bowel pain. Some women have endometriosis and these other pains. Migraine headaches are also common
❖ Women with chronic pain who appear "worn down" emotionally or depressed often have a neuropathic component to their pain. This will be worse if the patient is stressed or overworked
❖ Recognized that many women have had pain for long periods of time, resulting in loss of confidence, employment and education opportunities, relationship, and sometimes fertility
❖ It is important that the patient's family value her health and happiness, and that she has activities in her life that bring her joy, relaxation and satisfaction, fit, happy people have less pain
❖ Recognized that while surgery can be very helpful, it does not cure all pain. The decision whether to proceed to surgery or use nonsurgical treatment will depend on the surgical facilities available
❖ Be careful to explain the pain to the patient and make sure she knows that you believe in her pain. Most women with this type of pain have been told that "it is all in their head" which lowers their self-esteem
❖ Make sure that the family knows that the pain is real. The patient will need the support of her family to access care.

Surgical Intervention

When infertility is not a factor and the patient present with dysmenorrhea and/or dyspareunia, the medical approach may be provided prior to diagnostic surgery. However, after drug therapy the if the patient experiences a progression of the disease as determined with pelvic examination and/or ultrasound, or remains symptomatic, then operative intervention may be required. Prior to drug therapy for infertility, in light of the fact that medication is expensive, that there are side-effects and that pregnancy should be prevented while on such drug regimes, it is beneficial to confirm the diagnosis is endometriosis. Further, it is important to stage the disease in order to prescribe the appropriate modality of therapy. And the most efficacious method of diagnosis and staging endometriosis is with laparoscopy.

Through the laparoscope, not only can endometrial lesions be identified, but endometriotic areas can be fulgurated (burned) and adhesions lysed. With the addition of laser, through the laparoscope even extensive endometriotic tissue can be vaporized and adhesions removed. Furthermore, laparoscopic uterine nerve ablation, (LUNA) and subsequent nerve interrupting surgery has been the most effective modalities for relief of pain sans hysterectomy since we first performed the procedure in 1982. The laser vaporization of lesions at the time of laparoscopy affords the physician a means of treatment at the time of diagnosis. In fact, in hundred of my patients, laser laparoscopy has become the primary mode of therapy.

Surgical Technique

Routine preparation was made for diagnostic laparoscopy. With the patient intubated and under general anesthesia, the operating laparoscope was used to allow improved visualization and instrumentation of the cul de sac. LUNA surgery was then initiated. In the nulliparous the uterosacral ligaments were easily identified. Care was taken to avoid lateral pelvic structures, including the ureters. The operator stretched the uterosacral ligaments by flexing the uterus upwards toward the anterior abdominal wall. Next, using a generator (Medical electronics systems, model 2000) set at 5.8 W, the ligaments were coagulated at their insertion into the cervix using a 51 cm grasping forceps. Current was continued until blanching of the uterosacrals was noted. The effect on the tissue was limited to the uterosacral ligaments and slightly lateral. After desiccation the grasping forceps were used to connect the cauterized areas in a U-like fashion along the base of the cervix. Using the mechanical operating scissors, the uterosacral ligaments were cut through. Current was then reapplied to the depth of this incision. Cervical dilatation was not performed since it can bring temporary relief to the dysmenorrheic patient.

Laparoscopic Uterosacral Nerve Ablation

Laparoscopic uterosacral nerve ablation (LUNA) is a technique designed to disrupt the efferent nerve fibers in the uterosacral ligaments to decrease uterine pain for women with intractable dysmenorrhea. However, a large randomized controlled trail comparing results of conservative laparoscopic surgery for endometriosis to conservative surgery with LUNA observed no difference between groups in the proportions of patients having recurrent dysmenorrhea one and three years following surgery. Currently, LUNA does not appear to offer any added benefits beyond those that can be achieved with conservative surgery alone. Although LUNA has a low-risk of complications, uterine prolapsed and transection of the ureters can do occur.

In skilled hands, the risks of LUNA or laser surgery can be less than conventional 'open' incisions. LUNA research confirmed that the transection of the uterosacral nerves has its only action by releasing the uterine spasm and allowing the menstrual blood to egress more quickly. Whether the surgeon relies on LUNA or presacral neurectomy, the procedure has a 50 to 70% success at relieving painful menstrual periods.

Presacral Neurectomy

Presacral neurectomy involves interrupting the sympathetic innervations to the uterus at the level of the superior hypogastric plexus. One randomized controlled trial involving 71 women demonstrated that presacral neurectomy at time of conservative surgery for endometriosis decreased midline dysmenorrhea but did not improve other symptoms of dysmenorrhea dyspareunia, or pelvic pain. Another randomized controlled trial involving 141 women that compared results achieved with conservative laparoscopic surgery for endometriosis, with and without presacral neurectomy, observed that women treated by presacral neurectomy experienced significantly greater improvements in symptoms of dysmenorrhea dyspareunia, and pelvic pain between 6 to 12 months after surgery, compared with women treated by conservative surgery alone. Presacral neurectomy has been proposed for treatment of midline pain associated with menses, because its effects on other components of pelvic pain have been inconsistent. However, it is important to recognize that presacral neurectomy is a technically challenging procedure associated with significant risk of bleeding from the adjacent venous plexus. Success of this approach is debulking of the disease and the resulting surgical menopause causing atrophy of endometrial tissue. Hysterectomy without bilateral salpingooophorectomy is less effective, as disease recurrence and subsequent re-operation rates are higher.

Medical management of menopausal symptoms with hormone replacement following bilateral salpingo-oophorectomy carries the risk of recurrence of endometriosis and associated pain, and should be used with caution. Unopposed estrogen may be more likely to promote growth of endometriosis and disease recurrence than combined estrogen progestogen regimens, but no studies have compared the two treatments directly. In one randomized trial involving 175 women treated by TAH-BSO for endometriosis, the incidence of recurrent disease after a mean 46 months of follow-up in those who subsequently received cyclic estrogen and progestogen replacement was relatively low (3.5%), compared with untreated controls. Continuous combined estrogen-progestogen therapy is the recommended regimen for treating menopausal symptoms in women with endometriosis, an exception to the usual recommendation for estrogen only treatment after hysterectomy.

➲ MEDICAL THERAPY FOLLOWING CONSERVATIVE SURGERY FOR ENDOMETRIOSIS

Several studies have investigated the value of post-operative medical theapy. One prospective study found that, compared with placebo, six months of treatment with a GnRH agonist (Nafarelin acetate) after laparoscopic surgery for endometriosis resulted in greater improvement in pelvic pain and a longer interval before further treatment was required. In a larger study involving 269 women treated for six months with a GnRH agonist (Goserelin acetate) or placebo after aggressive surgical resection, postoperative medical treatment did not achieve significantly greater improvement in pain symptoms after one and two years of follow-up, although there was a strong trend in that direction. In a small randomized, controlled trial, treatment with danazol or MPA for six months following laparoscopy resulted in significantly more pain relief and reduction in the size of endometriotic lesions than placebo at the time of second look laparoscopy. No studies have evaluated postoperative therapy using less costly or intrusive treatments, such as cyclic or continuous OCs, or continuous progestogen treatment.

⟳ LONG-TERM MANAGEMENT

Endometriosis potentially is a chronic disease that can result in significant morbidity. Consequently, a long-term management plan would be beneficial. Endometriosis is viewed best primarily as a medical disease with surgical backup. Individuals with chronic superficial or presumed disease should be treated medically, reserving surgery for those having large endometriomas or palpable disease that fails to respond to treatment. For women diagnosed with endometriosis in the past, and those with recurrent symptoms, medical management again is the preferred approach. In such women, and in those who fail to respond to medical therapy, other causes of pelvic pain should be carefully considered before attributing the symptoms to endometriosis. Multiple surgical procedures should be avoided whenever possible, because surgery has inherent risks and also might result in adhesions that can cause pelvic pain. Women of reproductive age with endometriosis should be encouraged to pursue pregnancy at the earliest time that life circumstances allow because their disease has the potential to threaten their fertility.

⟳ SUMMARY AND CONCLUSION

❖ Endometriosis should be viewed as a chronic disease that requires a life-long management plan with the goal of maximizing the use of medical treatment and avoided repeated surgical procedures
❖ Gastrointestinal, urinary, musculoskeletal and psychological conditions can mimic the symptoms of endometriosis and should be excluded before pursuing aggressive therapy for endometriosis in all patients, particularly those who fail to respond to standard medical treatments
❖ Theories to explain the pain associated with endometriosis include the actions of humoral factors, the effects of active bleedings from implants, and the irritation or invasion of pelvic floor nerves by infiltrating implants.
❖ Laparoscopy remains the cornerstone of accurate diagnosis of endometriosis
❖ Both medical and surgical treatments for endometriosis are effective

❖ In women with symptoms of pelvic pain, visible endometriosis observed during surgery should be treated
❖ Surgical treatment for endometriosis, followed by medical therapy, offers longer symptom relief than surgery alone
❖ Definitive treatment of endometriosis should be reserved for women with debilitating symptoms that can reasonably be attributed to the disease who have completed childbearing and have failed to respond to alternative treatments
❖ Further studies designed to compare medical and surgical treatments are clearly warranted.

⇆ BIBLIOGRAPHY

1. Abbott J, Hawe J, Hunter D, Holmes M, Finn P, Garry R. Laparoscopic excision of endometriosis: a randomized, placebo-controlled trial. Fertil Steril. 2004;82:878–84.
2. Abbott JA, Hawe J, Clay ton RD, Garry R. The effects and effectiveness of laparoscopic excision of endometriosis: a prospective study with 2–5 years follow-up. Hum Reprod. 2003;18:1922–7.
3. Ailawadi RK, Jobanputra S, Kataria M, Gurates B, Bulun SE. Treatment of endometriosis and chronic pelvic pain with letrozole and norethindrone acetate: a pilot study. Fertil Steril. 2004;81:290–6.
4. Alborzi S, Momtahan M, Parsanezhad ME, Dehbashi S, Zolghadri J. A prospective, randomized study comparing laparoscopic ovarian cystectomy versus fenestration and coagulation in patients with endometriomas. Fertil Steril. 2004;82:1633–7.
5. Al-Jefout M, Palmer J, Fraser IS. Simultaneous use of a levonorgestrel intrauterine system and an etonogestrel subdermal implant for debilitating adolescent endometriosis. Aust N Z J Obstet Gynaecol. 2007;47:247–9.
6. American Society for Reproductive Medicine (ASRM). Revised American Society for Reproductive Medicine classification of endometriosis:1996. Fertil Steril. 1997;67:817–21.
7. Amster dam LL, Gentry W, Jobanputra S, Wolf M, Rubin SD, Bulun SE. Anastrazole and oral contraceptives: a novel treatment for endometriosis. Fertil Steril. 2005;84:300–4.
8. Arruda MS, Petta CA, Abrao MS, Benetti-Pinto CL. Time elapsed from onset of symptoms to diagnosis of endometriosis in a cohort study of Brazilian women. Hum Reprod. 2003;18:756–9.
9. Ballweg ML. Big picture of endometriosis helps provide guidance on approach to teens: comparative historical data show endo starting younger is more severe. J Pediatr Adolesc Gynecol. 2003;16(3):S21–6.
10. Barbieri RL. Hormone treament of endometriosis: the estrogen thresh old hypothesis. Am J Obstet Gynecol. 1992;166:740–5.
11. Barnhart K, Dunsmoor-Su R, Coutifaris C. Effect of endometriosis on in vitro fertilization. Fertil Steril. 2002;77:1148–55.
12. Bedaiwy MA, Casper RF. Treatment with leuprolide acetate and hormonal add-back for up to 10 years in stage IV endometriosis patients with chronic pelvic pain. Fertil Steril. 2006;86:220–2.
13. Behamondes L, Petta CA, Fernandes A, Monteiro I. Use of levonogesterol releasing intrauterine system in women with endometriosis, chronic pelvic pain and dysmenorrhea. Contraception. 2007;75(6):S134–9.

14. Beretta P, Franchi M, Ghezzi F, Busacca M, Zupi E, Bolis P. Randomized clinical trial of two laparoscopic treatments of endometriomas: cystectomy versus drainage and coagulation. Fertil Steril. 1998:70:1176–80.
15. Borgfeldt C, Andolf E. Cancer risk after hospital discharge diagnosis of benign ovarian cysts and endometriosis. Acta Obstet Gynecol Scand. 2004;83:395–400.
16. Brinton LA, Gridley G, Persson I, Baron J, Bergqvist A. Cancer risk after a hospital discharge diagnosis of endometriosis. Am J Obstet Gynecol. 1997;176:572–9.
17. Brinton LA, Sakoda LC, Sherman ME, Frederiksen K, Kjaer SK, Graubard BI, et al. Relationship of benign gynecologic diseases to subsequent risk of ovarian and uterine tumors. Cancer Epidemiol Biomarkers Prev. 2005;14:2929–35.
18. Bulun SE, Zeitoun KM, Takayama K, Sasano H. Estrogen biosynthesis in endometriosis: molecular basis and clinical relevance. J Mol Endocrinol. 2000;25(1): 35–42.
19. Bulun SE. Endometriosis. N Engl J Med. 2009;360:268–79.
20. Candiani GB, Fedele L, Candiani M. Double uterus, blind hemivagina, and ipsilateral renal agenesis: 36 cases and long-term follow-up. Obstet Gynecol. 1997;90:26–32.
21. Candiani GB, Fedele L, Vercellini P, Bianchi S, Di Nola G. Presacral neurectomy for the treatment of pelvic pain associated with endometriosis: 1. Fuller J, Ashar BS, Carey-Corrado J. Trocar-associated injuries and fatalities: an analysis of 1399 reports to the FDA. J Minim Invasive Gynecol. 2005;12:302–7.
22. Capron C, Fritel X, Dubuisson JB. Fertility after laparoscopic management of deep endometriosis infiltrating the uterosacral ligaments. Hum Reprod. 1999;14:329–32.
23. Casper RF. Estrogen with interrupted progestin HRT: a review of experimental and clinical studies. Maturitas. 2000;34:97–108.
24. Chapron C, Dubuisson JB. Laparoscopic treatment of deep endometriosis located on the uterosacral ligaments. Hum Reprod. 1996;11:868–73.
25. Chapron C, Fauconnier A, Goffinet F, Breart G, Dubuisson JB. Laparoscopic surgery is not inherently dangerous for patients presenting with benign gynecologic pathology: results of a meta-analysis. Hum Reprod. 2002;17:1334–42.
26. Chapron C, Pietin-Vialle C, Borghese B, Davy C, Foulot H, Cho pin N. Associated ovarian endometrioma is a marker for greater severity of deeply infiltrating endometriosis. Fertil Steril. 2009;92:453–7.
27. Chopin N, Vieira M, Borghese B, Foulot H, Dousset B, Coste J, et al. Operative management of deeply infiltrating endometriosis: results on pelvic pain symptoms according to a surgical classification. J Minim Invasive Gynecol. 2005;12:106–12.
28. Coffee AL, Sulai PJ, Kuehl TJ. Long-term assessment of symptomatology and satisfaction of an extended oral contraceptive regimen. Contraception. 2007;75:444–9.
29. Cornillie FJ, Oosterlynck D, Lauweryns JM, Konickx PR. Deeply infiltrating pelvic endometriosis: histology and clinical significance. Fertil Steril 1990;53:978–83.
30. Cosson M, Querleu D, Donnez J, Madelenat P, Konickx P, Audebert A, et al. Dienogest is as effective as triptorelin in the treatment of endometriosis after laparoscopic surgery: results of a prospective, multicenter, randomized study. Fertil Steril. 2002;77:684–92.
31. Cottrean CM, Ness RB, Moduqno F, Allen GO, Goodman MT. Endometriosis and its treatment with danazol or lupron in relation to ovarian cancer. Clin Cancer Res. 2003;9(14):5142–4.
32. Cottreau CM, Ness RB, Modugno F, Allen GO, Good man MT. Endometriosis and its treatment with danazol or lupron in relation.
33. Crosignani PG, Luciano A, Ray A, Bergqvist A. Subcutaneous depot medroxyprogesterone acetate versus leuprolide acetate in the treatment of endometriosis-associated pain. Hum Reprod. 2006;21:248–56.

34. Crosignani PG, Vercellini P, Biffignandi F, et al. Laparoscopy versus laparotomy in conservative surgical treatment for severe endometriosis. Fertil Steril. 1996;66:706–11.
35. D'Hooghe T, Debrock S, Hill JA, Mauleman C. Endometriosis and subfertility: is the relationship resolved? Semin Reprod Med. 2003:21:243-54.
36. Daniels J, Gray R, Hills RK, Lathe P, Buckley L, Gupta J, et al. LUND trial collaboration. Laparoscopic uterosacral nerve ablation for alleviating chronic pelvic pain: a randomized controlled trial. JAMA. 2009;302:955–61.
37. Darai E, Bazot M, Rouzier R, Houry S, Dubernard G. Outcome of laparoscopic colorectal resection for endometriosis. Curr Opin Obstet Gynecol. 2007;19:308–13. Acta Obstet Gynecol Scand Suppl 1994. Fertil Steril 1998;70:1101.
38. Davis AR, Westhoff C, O'Connell K, Gallagher N. Oral contraceptives for dysmenorrhea in adolescent girls. Obstet Gynecol. 2005;106:97–104.
39. Davis GD, Thillet E, Lindemann J. Clinical characteristics of adolescent endo-metriosis. J Adolesc Health. 1993;14:362–8.
40. DeWilde RL, Trew RG. Postoperative abdominal adhesions and their prevention in gynaeco logical surgery. Expert consensus position. Part 2–steps to reduce adhesions. Gynecol Surg. 2007;4:243–53.
41. DiVasta AD, Laufer MR, Gordon C. Bone density in adolescent treated with a GnRH agonist and add-back therapy for endometriosis. J Pediatr Adolesc Gynecol. 2007;20:293–7.
42. Dmowksi WP, Scholer HF, Mahesh VB, Greenblatt RB. Danazol — a synthetic steroid derivative with interesting physiologic properties. Fertil Steril. 1971;22:9–18.
43. Donnez J, Nisolle-Pochet M, Clerckx-Braun F, Sandow J, Casanas-Roux F. Administration of nasal buserelin as compared wlth subcutaneous buserelin implant for endometriosis. Fertil Steril. 1989;52:27–30.
44. Emmert C, Romann D, Riedel HH. Endometriosis diagnosed by laparoscopy in adolescent girls. Arch Gynecol Obstet. 1998;261:89–93.
45. Fauconnier A, Chapron C. Endometriosis and pelvic pain: epidemiological evidence of the relationship
46. Fedele L, Bianchi S, Zanconato G, Portuese A, Raffaelli R. Use of a levonorgestrel-releasing intrauterine device in the treatment of rectovaginal endometriosis. Fertil Steril. 2001;75:485–8.
47. Feeley KM, Wells M. Precursor lesions of ovarian epithelial malignancy. Histo-pathology. 2001;38:87–95.
48. Frishman GN, Salak JR. Conservative surgical management of endometriosis in women with pelvic pain. J Minim Invasive Gynecol. 2006;13:546–58.
49. Giudice LC, Kao LC. Endometriosis. Lancet. 2004;364:1789–99.
50. Goldstein DP, De Cholnoky C, Emans SJ. Adolescent endometriosis. J Adolesc Health Care. 1980;1:37–41.
51. Gover S. Pelvic pain in the female adolescent. Aust Fam Physician. 2006;35:850–3.
52. Greco D. Management of adolescent chronic pelvic pain from endometriosis: a pain center perspective. J Pediatr Adolesc Gynecol. 2003;16(3 Suppl):S17–9
53. Had field R, Mardon H, Barlow D, Kennedy S. Delay in the diagnosis of endometriosis: a survey of women from the USA and UK. Hum Reprod. 1996;11:878–80.
54. Harada T, Momoeda M, Taketani Y, Aso T, Fukunaga M, Hagino H, et al. Dienogest is as effective as intranasal buserelin acetate for the relief of pain symptoms associated with endometriosis—a randomized, double-blind, multicenter, controlled trial. Fertil Steril. 2009
55. Harada T, Momoeda M, Taketani Y, Hiroshi H, Terakawa N. Low-dose oral contraceptive pill for dysmenorrhea associated with endometriosis: a placebo-controlled, double-blind, randomized trial. Fertil Steril. 2008;90:1583–8.

56. Harel Z. A contemporary approach to dysmenorrhea in adolescents. Pediatr Drugs. 2002;4:797–805.
57. Hart RJ, Hickey M, Maouris P, Buckett W. Excisional surgery versus ablative surgery for ovarian endometriomata. Cochrane Data base Syst Rev. 2008;16(2):CD004992.
58. Higgins MJ, Davidson NE. What is the current status of ovarian suppression/ablation in women with premenopausal early-stage breast cancer? Curr Oncol Rep. 2009;11:45–50.
59. Hornstein MD, Surrey ES, Weisberg GW, Casino LA. Leuprolide acetate depot and hormonal add-back in endometriosis: a 12-month study. Lupron Add-Back Study Group. Obstet Gynecol. 1998;91:16–24.
60. Hughes E, Brown J, Collins JJ, Farquhar C, Fedorkow DM, Vandekerckhove P. Ovulation suppression for endometriosis. Cochrane Data base Syst Rev. 2007 18;(3):CD000155.
61. Husby GK, Haugen RS, Moen MH. Diagnostic delay in women with pain and endometriosis. Acta Obstet Gynecol Scand. 2003.
62. Jain S, Dal ton ME. Chocolate cysts from ovarian follicles. Fertil Steril. 1999;72:852–6.
63. Jansen RP. Minimal endometriosis and reduced fecundability: prospective evidence from an artificial insemination by donor program. Fertil Steril. 1986;46(1):141–3.
64. Jarrell JF, Vilos GA, Allaire C, Burgess S, Fortin C, Gerwin R. Chronic Pelvic Pain Committee. Consensus guidelines for the management of chronic pelvic pain, part 1. SOGC Clinical Practice Guideline No. 164, August 2005. J Obstet Gynaecol Can. 2005
65. Jenkins TR, Liu CY, White J. Does response to hormonal therapy predict presence or absence of endometriosis? J Minim Invasive gynecol. 2008;15:82–6.
66. Jones KD, Haines P, Sutton CJ. Long-term follow-up of a controlled trial of laser laparoscopy for pelvic pain. JSLS. 2001;5:111–5.
67. Kobayashi H, Sumimoto K, Moniwa N, et al. Risk of developing ovarian cancer among women with ovarian endometrioma: a cohort study in Shizuoka, Japan. Int J Gynecol Can cer. 2007;17:37–43.
68. Koga K, Takemura Y, Osuga Y, Yoshino O, Hirota Y, Hirata T, et al. Recurrence of ovarian endometrioma after laparoscopic excision. Hum Reprod. 2006;21:2171–4.
69. Koninckx PR, Meuleman C, Oosterlynck D, Cornillie FJ. Diagnosis of deep endometriosis by clinical examination during menstruation and plasma CA-125 concentration. Fertil Steril. 1996;65:280–7.
70. Laufer MR, Goietein L, Bush M, Cramer DW, Emans SJ. Prevalence of endometriosis in adolescent girls with chronic pelvic pain not responding to conventional therapy. J Pediatr Adolesc Gynecol. 1997;10:199–202.
71. Le T, Giede C, Salem S. SOGC/GOC/SCC Policy and Practice Guidelines Committee. Initial evaluation and referral guidelines for management of pelvic/ovarian masses. Joint SOGC/GOC/SCC clinical practice guideline No. 230, 2009. J Obstet Gynaecol Can. 2009;31:668–73.
72. Le T, Giede C. SOGC/GOC/SCC Policy and Practice Guidelines Committee. Initial evaluation and referral guidelines for management of pelvic/ovarian masses. SOGC Joint Clinical Practice Guide line, No. 230, 2009. J Obstet Gynaecol Can 2009;31:668cer 2006; 119:556ween endometriosis and cancer: a comprehensive review.
73. Lichten, EM. Surgical Treatment of primary dysmenorrhea: Laparoscopic uterine nerve ablation (LUNA). J Reproductive Medicine. 1987;32(1):37-41.
74. Littman E, Giudice L, Lathi R, Berker B, Milki A, Nezhat C. Role of laparoscopic treatment of endometriosis in patients with failed in vitro fertilization cycles. Fertil Steril. 2005;84:1574–8.

75. Lower AM, Haw thorn RJ, Ellis H, O'Brien F, Buchan S, Crowe AM. The impact of adhesions on hospital readmissions over ten years after 8849 open gynaecological operations: an assessment from the surgical and clinical adhesions research study. Br J Obstet Gynaecol 2000;107:855–62. a controlled study. Am J Obstet Gynecol. 1992;167:100–3.

76. Marcoux S, Maheux R, Bérubé S. Canadian Collaborative Group on Endometriosis. Laparoscopic surgery in infertile women with minimal or mild endometriosis. N Engl J Med. 1997;337:217–22.

77. Marsh EE, Laufer MR. Endometriosis in premenarcheal girls who do not have an associated obstructed anomaly. Fertil Steril. 2005;83:758–60.

78. Matsuzaki S, Houlle C, Darcha C, Pouly JL, Mage G, Canis M. Analysis of risk factors for the removal of normal ovarian tissue during laparoscopic cystectomy for ovarian endometriosis. Hum Reprod. 2009;24:1402–6.

79. Melin A, Sparen P, Persson I, Bergqvist A. Endometriosis and the risk of cancer with special emphasis on ovarian cancer. Hum Reprod. 2006;21:1237–42.

80. Mereu L, Ruffo G, Landi S, Barbieri F, Zaccoletti R, Fiaccavento A, et al. Laparoscopic treatment of deep endometriosis with segmental colorectal resection: short term morbidity. J Minim Invasive Gynecol. 2007;14:463–9.

81. Milburn A, Reiter RC, Rhomberg AT. Multidisciplinary approach to chronic pelvic pain. Obstet Gynecol Clin North Am. 1993;20:643–61.

82. Mitwally MF, Gotlieb L, Ca per RF. Prevention of bone loss and hypoestrogenic symptoms by estrogen and interrupted progestogen add-back in long-term GnRH-agonist down-related patients with endometriosis and premenstrual syndrome. Menopause. 2002;9:236–41.

83. Mol BW, Bayram N, Lijmer JG, Wiegerinck MA, Bongers MY, vander Veen F, et al. The performance of CA-125 measurement in the detection

84. Muneyyirci-Delate O, Karacan M. Effect of norethindrone acetate in the treatment of symptomatic endometriosis. Int J Fertil Womens Med. 1998;43:24–7.

85. Ness RB, Cramer DW, Good man MT, Kjaer SK, Mallin K, Mosgaard BJ, et al. Infertiity, fertility drugs, and ovarian cancer: a pooled analysis of case-control studies. Am J Epidemiol. 2002;155:217–24.

86. Nezhat F, Datta MS, Hanson V, Pejovic T, Nezhat C, Nezhat C. The relationship of endometriosis and ovarian malignancy: a review. Fertil Steril. 2008;90:1559–70.

87. Ogawa S, Kaku T, Amada S, Kobayashi H, Hirakawa T, Ariyoshi K, et al. Ovarian endometriosis associated with ovarian carcinoma: a clinicopathological and immunohistochemical study. Gynecol Oncol. 2000;77:298–304.

88. Olive D, Henderson D. Endometrosis and Müllerian anomalies. Obstet Gynecol. 1987;69:412–5.

89. Olson JE, Cerhan JR, Janney CA, Anderson KE, Vachon CM, Sellers TA. Postmenopausal cancer risk after self-reported endometriosis diagnosis in the Iowa women's health study. Cancer. 2002;94:1612–8.

90. Oral E, Ilvan S, Tustas E, Korbeyli B, Bese T, Demirkiran F, et al. Prevalence of endometriosis in malignant epithelial ovary tumours. Eur J Obstet Gynecol Reprod Biol. 2003;109:97–101.

91. Otsuka J, Okuda T, Sekizawa A, Amemiya S, Saito H, Okai T, et al. K-ras mutation may pro mote carcinogenesis of endometriosis leading to ovarian clear cell carcinoma. Med Electron Microsc. 2004;37:188–92.

92. Packard CJ, Shep herd J. Action of danazol on plasma lipids and lipoprotein.

93. Parazzini F. Ablation of lesions or no treatment in minimal–mild endometriosis in infertile women: a randomized trial. Gruppo Italiano perlo St dio dell'Endometriosis. Hum Reprod. 1999;14:1332–4.

94. Petta CA, Ferriani RA, Abrao MS, Hassan D, Rosa E Silva JC, et al. Randomized clinical trial of a levonorgestrel-releasing intrauterine system and a depot GnRH analogue for the treatment of chronic pelvic pain in women with endometriosis. Hum Reprod. 2005;20:1993–8.

95. Progesterone resistance in endometriosis: link to failure to metabolise. Mol Cell Endocrinol. 2006;248:94–103.

96. Progesterone resistance in endometriosis: link to failure to metabolize estradiol. Mol Cell Endocrinol. 2006;248:94–103.

97. Prowse AH, Manek S, Varma R, Liu J, Godwin AK, Maher ER, et al. Molecular genetic evidence that endometriosis is a precursor of ovarian cancer. Int J Can.

98. Rana N, Thomas S, Rotman C, Dmowski WP. Decrease in the size of ovarian endometriomas during ovarian suppression in stage IV endometriosis. Role of pre operative medical treatment. J Reprod Med. 1996;41:384–92.

99. Rawson JM. Prevalence of endometriosis in asymptomatic women. J Reprod Med. 1991;36:513–5.

100. Razzi S, Luisi S, Calonaci F, Altomare A, Bocchi C, Patraglia F. Efficacy of vaginal danazol treatment in women with recurrent deeply infiltrating endometriosis. Fertil Steril. 2007:88:789–94.

101. Reese KA, Reddy S, Rock JA. Endometriosis in an adolescent population: the Emory experience. J Pediatr Adolesc Gynecol. 1996;9:125–8.

102. Rock JA, Breech LL. Surgery for anomalies of the Müllerian ducts. In: Rock JA, Jones HW, (eds) Te Linde's Operative gynecology. 9th edition Philadelphia: Lippincott Williams and Wilkins; 2003.

103. Royal College of Obstetricians and Gynaecologists. The investigation and management of endometriosis (green-top guideline; no. 24). London (England): RCOG;2006:3.

104. Sallam HN, Garcia-Velasco JA, Dias S, Arici A. Long-term pituitary down-regulation before in vitro fertilization (IVF) for women with endometriosis. Cochrane Data base Syst Rev. 2006,25(1):CD004635.

105. Sampson JA. Endometrial carcinoma of the ovary arising in endometrial tissue in that organ. Arch Surg. 1925;10:1–72.

106. Sampson JA. Peritoneal endometriosis due to menstrual dissemination of endo-metrial tissue into the peritoneal cavity. Am J Obstet Gynecol. 1927;14:422–69.

107. Sanfilippo J, Wakim N, Schikler K, Yussman M. Endometriosis in association with uterine anomaly. Am J Obstet Gynecol. 1986;154:39–43.

108. Sasagawa S, Shimizu Y, Kami H, Takeuchi T, Mita S, Imada K, et al. Dienogest is a selective progesterone receptor agonist in transactivation analysis with potent oral endometrial activity due to its efficient pharmacokinetic profile. Steroids. 2008;73:222–31.

109. Scarselli G, Rizzello F, Cammilli F, Ginocchini L, Coccia ME. Diagnosis and treatment of endometriosis. A review. Minerva Ginecol. 2005;57:55–78.

110. Schlaff WD, Car son SA, Luciano A, Ross D, Bergqvist A. Subcutaneous injection of depot medroxyprogesterone acetate compared with leuprolide acetate in the treatment of endometriosis-associated pain. Fertil Steril. 2006;85:314–25.

111. Schwartz D, Mayaux MJ. Female fecundity as a function of age: results of artificial insemination in 2193 nulliparous women with azoospermic husbands. Federation CECOS. N Engl J Med 1982;307:404–6.

112. Scott RB. Malignant changes in endometriosis. Obstet Gynecol. 1953;2:283–9.

113. Selak V, Farquhar C, Prentice A, Singla A. Danazol for pelvic pain associated with endometriosis. Cochrane Data base Syst Rev. 2007;(4):CD000068.

114. Seracchioli R, Mabrouk M, Frascà C, Manuzzi L, Savelli L, Venturoli S. Long-term oral contraceptive pills and postoperative pain management after laparoscopic excision of ovarian endometrioma: a randomized controlled trial. Fertil Steril. 2009.

115. Seracchioli R, Mabrouk M, Manuzzi L, Vicenzi C, Frascà C, Elmakky A, et al. Postoperative use of oral contraceptive pills for prevention of anatomical relapse or symptom-recurrence after conservative surgery for endometriosis. Hum Reprod. 2009;24:2729–35.

116. Shakiba K, Bena JF, McGill KM, Minger J, Falcone T. Surgical treatment of endometriosis: a 7-year follow-up on the requirement for further surgery. Obstet Gynecol. 2008;111:1285–92. Erratum in: Obstet Gynecol 2008;112:710.

117. Singh SS, Marcoux V, Cheung V, Mar tin D, Ternamian AM. Core competencies for gynecologic endoscopy in residency training: a national consensus project. J Minim Invasive Gynecol. 2009;16(1):1–7.

118. Somigliana E, Vercellini P, Viganó P, Ragni G, Crosignani PG. Should endometriomas be treated before IVF-ICSI cycles? Hum Reprod. 2006;21:57–64.

119. Somigliana E, Vigano P, Parazzini F, Stoppelli S, Giambattista E, Vercellini P. Association betand a critical analysis of clinical and epidemiological evidence. Gynecol Oncol. 2006;101:331–41.

120. Stavroulis AI, Saridogan E, Creigh ton SM, Cutner AS. Laparoscopic treatment of endometriosis in teenagers. Eur J Obstet Gynecol Reprod Biol. 2006;248–50.

121. Strowitzki T, Marr J, Gerlinger C, Faustmann T, Seitz C. Dienogest is as effective as leuprolide acetate in treating the painful symptoms of endometriosis: a 24-week, randomized, multicentre, open-label trial. Hum Reprod. 2010;25:633–41.

122. Strowitzki T, Seitz C, Marr J, Gerlinger C, Faustmann 1. Efficacy of dienogest for the treatment of endometriosis: a 24-week, randomised, open-label trial versus leuprolide acetate. Abstract presented at: 25th Annual Meeting of the European Society of Human Reproduction and Embryology; Amsterdam; 2009.

123. Surrey ES, Hornstein MD. Prolonged GnRH agonist and add-back therapy for symptomatic endometriosis: long-term follow-up. Obstet Gynecol. 2002;99(51): 709–19.

124. Sutton CJ, Ewan SP, Whitelaw N, Haines P. Prospective, randomized,double-blind, controlled trial of laser laparoscopy in the treatment of pelvic pain associated with minimal, mild, and moderate endometriosis. Fertil Steril. 1994;62:696–700.

125. Templeman C. Adolescent endometriosis. Obstet Gynecol Clin North Am. 2009;36:177–86.

126. The journal of the American Board of Family Medicine. 2004;17

127. Tummon IS, Asher LJ, Mar tin JS, Tulandi T. Randomized controlled trial of superovulation and insemination for infertility associated with minimal or mild endometriosis. Fertil Steril. 1997;68:8–12.

128. Valenzuela P, Ramos P, Redondo S, Cabrera Y, Alvarez I, Ruiz A. Endometrioid adenocarcinoma of the ovary and endometriosis. Eur J Obstet Gynecol Reprod Biol. 2007; 34:83–6.

129. Van Gorp T, Amant F, Neven P, Vergote I, Moerman P. Endometriosis and the development of malignant tumours of the pelvis. A review of literature. Best Pract Res Clin Obstet Gynaecol 2004;18:349–71.

130. Varma R, Rollason T, Gupta JK, Maher ER. Endometriosis and the neoplastic process. Reproduction. 2004;127:293–304.

131. Vercellini P, Aimi G, Panazza S, De Giorgi O, Pesole A, Crosignani PG. A levonorgestrel-releasing intrauterine system for the treatment of dysmenorrhea associated with endometriosis: a pilot study. Fertil Steril. 1999;72:505–8.

132. Vercellini P, Fedele L, Arcaini L, Bianchi S, Rognoni M, Candiani G. Laparoscopy in the diagnosis of chronic pelvic pain in adolescent women. J Reprod Med. 1989;34:827–30.
133. Vercellini P, Frontino G, De Giorgi O, Pietropaolo G, Pasin R, Crosignani PG. Continuous use of an oral contraceptive for endometriosis-associated recurrent dysmenorrhea that does not respond to a cyclic pill regimen. Fertil Steril. 2003;80: 560–3.
134. Vigano P, Somigliana E, Parazzini F, Vercellini P. Bias versus causality: interpreting recent evidence of association between endometriosis and ovarian cancer. Fertil Steril. 2007;88:588–93.
135. Waller KG, Lindsay P, Curtis P, Shaw RW. The prevalence of endometriosis in women with infertile partners. Eur J Obstet Gynecol Reprod Biol. 1993;48:135–9.
136. Wayne PM, Kerr CE, Schnyer RN, Legedza ATR, Savetsky-Ger man J, Shields MH, et al. Japanese-style acupuncture for endometriosis-related pelvic pain in adolescents and young women: results of a randomized controlled trial. J Pediatr Adolesc Gynecol. 2008;21:247–5.
137. Wheeler JM. Epidemiology and prevalence of endometriosis. Infertil Reprod Med Clin North Am. 1992;3:545–9.
138. Wie HJ, Lee JH, Kyung MS, Jung US, Choi JS. Is incidental appendectomy necessary in women with ovarian endometrioma? Aust N Z J Obstet Gynaecol. 2008;48: 107–111.
139. Winkel CA. Evaluation and management of women with endometriosis. Obstet Gynecol. 2003;102:397–408.
140. Woolf SH, Battista RN, Angerson GM, Logan AG, Eel W. Canadian Task Force on Preventive Health Care. New grades for recommendations from the Canadian Task Force on Preventive Health Care. Can Med Assoc J. 2003;169(3):207-8.
141. Wright J, Lotfallah H, Jones K, Lovell D. A randomized trial of excision versus ablation for mild endometriosis. Fertil Steril. 2005;83:1830–6.
142. Zullo F, Palomba S, Zupi E, Russo T, Morelli M, Cappiello F, et al. Effectiveness of presacral neurectomy in women with severe dysmenorrheal caused by endometriosis who were treated with laparoscopic conservative surgery: a 1-year prospective randomized double-blind controlled trial. Am J Obstet Gynecol. 2003;189:5–10.
143. Zullo F, Palomba S, Zupi E, Russo T, Morelli M, Sena T, et al. Long-term effectiveness of presacral neurectomy for the treatment of severe dysmenorrhea due to endometriosis. J Am Assoc Gynecol Laparosc. 2004;11:23–8.
144. Zupi E, Marconi D, Sbracia M, Zullo F, De Vivo B, Exacustos C, et al. Add-back therapy in the treatment of endometriosis-associated pain. Fertil Steril. 2004;82:1303–8.

Recurrent Endometriosis: Clinicians Challenge

◀ Kanthi Bansal

The natural history of endometriosis, like the factors that influence its occurence and course,has still to be defined. On the other hand, its capacity to recur even after apparently adequate conservative surgery is well-known.

When symptoms of endometriosis reappear several months after treatment, it is difficult to distinguish between recurrence and persistence of the disease. Endometriosis is a condition which is not curable, therefore recurrence of this enigmatic disease is inevitable. The smaller and invisible implants are not removed during surgery and the medical management does not cure the entity, thus leading to recurrence.

○ PREVALENCE OF RECURRENCE

Endometriosis tends to recur after conservative surgery or medical treatment unless definitive surgery is performed.[1] Nevertheless, ambiguities regarding the natural history of endometriosis make the precise prediction of recurrence difficult. According to the prevalent theory, recurrence of endometriosis represents an evolution of lesions, which are invisible at the time of treatment or visible but subtle and therefore not taken into account in the treamnet process or, finally, result of incomplete surgical approach.[2] Recurrence rate varies among 5 to 20% per year, reaching 40 to 50%, five years after initial treatment. Additional studies suggest that the *ex novo* formation of endometriotic lesions accompanied by corresponding clinical manifestations.[3] It is known that no histological difference has been demonstrated between initial and recurrent endometriotic lesions.

The most frequent clinical presentations of endometriosis include dys-menorrhea, pelvic pain, dyspareunia, infertility, and pelvic mass. However, the correlation between these symptoms and the stage of endometriosis is poor. Currently available laboratory markers are of limited value. At present, the best marker, serum CA-125, is usually elevated only in advanced stages and therefore not suitable for routine screening. Transvaginal ultrasound and magnetic resonance imaging are often helpful, particularly in detection of endometriotic cysts. Recently, transrectal ultrasound and magnetic resonance imaging were shown to be valuable in detection of deep infiltrating lesions, especially in the rectovaginal septum.

⊃ CAUSES OF RECURRENCE

There has not been much study onto the apt causes of the recurrene of the dreadful disease. Several clinical studies suggest that the recurring endometriotic lesions arise from residual lesions or cells not completely removed during the primary surgery. Women who receive microsurgical resection of ovarian endometriosis, a high prevalence of active endometriosis without signs of degeneration is found after hormonal therapy.[4]

Hormonal treatment does not lead to a complete suppression of endometriotic foci and that recurring lesions appear to grow from the residual loci[5] found that for those patients who underwent a second surgery, the recurrence of deep endometriosis is observed in the 'same' area of the pelvis involved in the first operation. Administration of steroids also elicited regrowth of suppressed endometriosis previously suppressed by the Gn-RH agonist.[6] This resilience of endometriosis seems to be consistent with the treatment failure and recurrence of the disease in women.

There are studies to suggest that recurrence may originate from *de novo* lesions derived from endometrium through retrograde menstruation.

Laparoscopy plus laser ablation of endometrium effectively eliminated recurrence at least in the first 2 years after surgery.[7] This finding appears to provide a strong piece of evidence in support for a role of eutopic endometrium in recurrence, possibly through abnormal uterine contraction[8] and subsequent tubal dissemination of endometrial debris.

There is also a possibility that lymph node involvement by endometriotic foci and lymphovascular invasion could be responsible for recurrence. Lymph node involvement and lymphovascular invasion are frequently found in deep infiltrating rectosigmoid endometriosis and are correlated with the size of the lesions.[9] Lymph node involvement in some rare forms of endometriosis also has been reported.[10] Lymph node involvement may be indicative of an invasive process just like cancer metastasis, possibly responsible for recurrence. Alternatively, however, it may be due simply to lymphatic drainage from endometriotic tissues. In addition, whether some more common forms of deep infiltrating endometriosis also have lymph node involvement are unclear.

Immunological factors may also contribute to the recurrence of endometriosis.

It also has been reported that the estrogen receptor polymorphism estrogen receptor a-Pvull may be responsible for increased propensity to recurrence.[11]

Diagnosis of Recurrent Endometriosis

The longer that this disease goes undiagnosed the more damage it can do. There are several new and less invasive surgical method of diagnosing recurrent endometriosis.

Laparoscopy

The most reliable way to confirm the presence of the recurrence of the disease is by visually inspecting the abdominal organs by laparoscopy procedure **(Fig. 12.1)**. The recurrent endometrial growths can easily be seen. Because endometriosis implants or growths vary in appearance and can be mistaken for other conditions, the lesions should be surgically removed and examined under a microscope to confirm the recurrence of the disease.

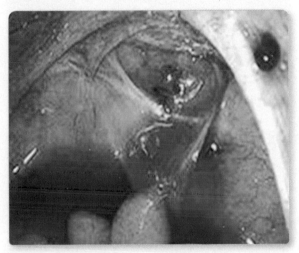

Figure 12.1: Recurrent endometrial implants

Imaging Tests

Imaging tests (e.g. pelvic ultrasound, magnetic resonance imaging) may be used to identify recurrence of individual endometrial lesions, but they are not used to determine the extent of the disease. The implants are not easily identified using this method **(Figs 12.2 and 12.3)**.

Biomarkers for Recurrence

The identification of biomarkers for recurrence, which so far has received little attention, may help illuminate the causes of recurrence. The identification of risk factors may promise to identify subpopulation of patients with high risk of recurrence and may possibly provide some insight as to why and how recurrence occurs, it should be noted that even if a risk factor is universally accepted, its power in predicting recurrence may be high in a population but low for a given patient. Without knowing the mechanisms of recurrence, there is simply nothing that can be done about certain putative risk factors, such as age at surgery and high rAFS scores, particularly so, given the limited effectiveness of current interventions.

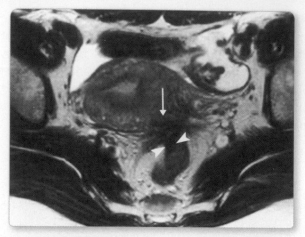

Figure 12.2: Recurrent endometrial lesion on MRI

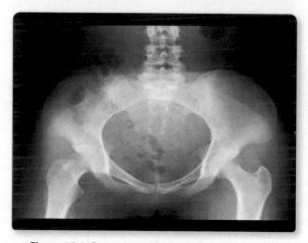

Figure 12.3: Recurrent endometrial implant on X-ray

A biomarker, which is a biochemical feature derived from the patient, is more likely to be individually specific since it can be used to characterize the progress of disease or the effects of treatment. Yet, it is somewhat surprising that very scant attention has been paid to the identification of reliable prognostic biomarkers, preferably available around the time of surgery, that are predictive of recurrence. The availability of these biomarkers would afford identification of patients with a high-risk of recurrence, potentially paving the way for intervention. Indeed, the identification of high-risk patients and targeted intervention, likely through pharmacological means, would be preferable to intervening indiscriminately. Since most, if not all, drugs have side effects, the targeted intervention might be more effective while reducing side effects and costs. The rapid advances in genomics, epigenomics and proteomics are opening up new avenues to the discovery of novel biomarkers for recurrence of endometriosis, as well as non-invasive diagnostic procedures.

COX-2 overexpression in ectopic endometrium taken at the time of surgery, along with previous medical treatment of endometriosis and the presence of adhesion, is predictive of recurrence of ovarian endometrioma within 30 months after surgery. COX-2 overexpression is associated with increased risk of recurrence of ovarian endometrioma strongly suggests that there are identifiable molecular genetic differences intrinsic to the lesion tissue samples, and these differences confer different risks for recurrence.

The finding that COX-2 overexpression, previous medical treatment of endometriosis and the presence of adhesions jointly constitute a modest predictor of recurrence is in broad agreement with the previous report that previous medical treatment of endometriosis is one of three risk factors for the recurrence of ovarian endometrioma.[12] However, with the introduction of COX-2 positivity as a biomarker, age at surgery and rAFS score were no longer associated with the recurrence risk. It is possible that COX-2 positivity, along with the presence of adhesion or not, may have captured the aggressiveness of the disease in terms of recurrence potential and completely eclipsed the predictive ability of rAFS score and other clinical variables.

Management of Recurrent Endometriosis

Management of endometriosis focuses on pain relief and includes medical and surgical treatment. Pharmacologic therapies currently in use include combination oral contraceptives (COCs), danazol, Gn-RH analogues and progestins. Although some agents show efficacy in relieving pain, all differ in their side effects, making it difficult to achieve a balance between efficacy and safety. Efficacy has been demonstrated with danazol or Gn-RH analogues; however, treatment is limited to 6 months because of significant metabolic side effects. Alternatives for longer-term management of symptoms include addback therapy with Gn-RH analogues, COCs or progestins. Newer options for treatment of endometriosis include depot medroxyprogesterone acetate subcutaneous injection. A very promising therapy is insertion of levonorgestrel-releasing intrauterine device (LNG-IUD),is useful in cases of recurrent endometriosis. There are several agents under investigation that may prove to have therapeutic potential. In women with recurrent endometriosis and recurrent pelvic pains, several options of treatment may be considered. Clinical response to prior surgery and medical treatments as well as frequency and intensity of side effects of these treatments should be the guidelines in treatment selection. If there was a good and lasting response after surgical resection, another laparoscopic surgery may be considered. It should, however, be kept in mind that repeated surgeries cause adhesions and destruction of healthy ovarian tissue and may adversely affect fertility.

Surgical Management

The availability of an efficacious and minimally invasive surgical technique makes the appropriateness of the current therapeutic alternatives for recurrent endometriosis highly controversial. It is currently believed that infertile women with recurrent endometriosis should be included in assisted reproduction programs. However, the poor results of these techniques and their cost make operative laparoscopy the treatment of choice in such women. Likewise, operative laparoscopy seems to offer notable advantages with respect to repeated courses of medical therapy which are necessary for patients with pelvic pain associated with recurrent endometriosis. Unfortunately, the effect of the pharmacological treatments now available usually disappears shortly after their suspension. In addition, these drugs may be expensive and have frequent adverse reactions. The definitive surgery is considered the treatment of choice for recurrence, a second conservative intervention is often preferred due to the patient's young age and her desire for children.

Operative laparoscopy is as efficacious in the treatment of recurrent endometriosis as it is in the treatment of the primary disease, and simplifies management of the disease for the clinician **(Fig. 12.4)**.

Laparoscopic treatment of endometriosis involves destroying the endo-metriotic lesions using electrosurgical desiccation or fulgration or by laser evaporation for minimal to mild disease while lysis of adhesions and excision of deep fibrotic lesions may have to be performed for more sever forms of the disease.

The laser and electrosurgery have the advantage of hemostasis but there is a risk of collateral damage. The newly invented technique of cavitational ultrasonic surgical aspirator (CUSA) using a probe with ultrasonic tip vibrating at 23 kHz causing emulsification of the cell membrane of the endometriotic

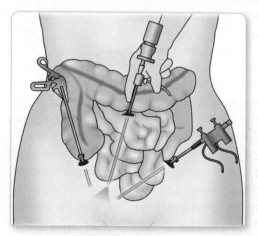

Figure 12.4: Operative laparoscopy

implants and adhesions which then irrigated to remove debris. It is claimed better visibility and helps to differentiate between target tissues. The relative efficacy has to be awaited. Laparoscopy assisted vaginal hysteroscopy (LAVH) or total laparoscopic hysterectomy (TLH) may have to be performed in intractable or recurrent disease. More recently laparoscopic pelvic peritoneal excision has been introduced as a way of preventing recurrence.

Laparotomy and nowadays laparoscopy, the latter currently the treatment of choice, are both used for used for managing endometriosis.[13] Therefore, re-operation is usually considered to be the best treatment option for recurrent disease in comparison with the hormonal therapy or expectant management, although its extent and duration of the effect are still unclear.[14] In patients with recurrent ovarian endometriosis, the impact of the surgical trauma on the reoperated ovary with a possible detrimental effect on its function and future folliculogenesis, should always be taken into account in the adoption of the preferred conservative laparoscopic method for the treatment of the endometriotic cysts.[15]

If there are chances of recurrence, techniques like meticulous excision of the implants, inspection and adhesiolysis in the pouch of Douglas, mobilization of the ovaries and tubes are considered. Extensive fibrosis is not uncommon in endometriosis recurrence, involving the peritoneum over the ureters setting great surgical difficulties even for the experienced surgeon. Under these circumstances ureteral stenosis can occur in 10% of cases with deep infiltrating implants larger tha 3 cm in size and therefore ureteral dissection is essential.[16]

Dissection of the ureter should be necessary in order to avoid injuries and severe complications. Laparoscopic uterine nerve ablation (LUNA) is an advanced procedure and should be reserved for patients with recurrent midline pain.

The role of transvaginal ultrasound (TVS) in the diagnosis of recurrent endometriosis, the authors concluded that endometriomas detected by ultrasound scan, may remain asymptomatic, therefore a second operation to treat these depends more on the presenting symptoms than on the endometrioma's size. Nevertheless, it is known that women suffering from severe pelvic pain usually have large endometriomas which are commonly accompanied by other endometriotic lesions such as deep nodules, adnexal and/or bowel adhesions. The latter patients require more frequently a second surgical intervention.

The recurrence rate of deep endometriosis after surgical removal of the nodule was 3.7% and resection of the posterior vaginal fornix, while this percentage was 16%, when vaginal fornix resection was not performed and raised up to 20%, when the bowel alone was resected without the vaginal fornix and conservation of the rectum.

➲ POSTOPERATIVE MEDICAL MANAGEMENT IN RECURRENT ENDOMETRIOSIS

All three major classes of medication in treating endometriosis, namely, progestins, Gn-RH agonists and androgenic agents such as danazol, suppress proliferation of the implants and reduce adhesion formation.[17] It appears to be sensible to treat patients with endometriosis postoperatively in the hope to eliminate residual endometriotic cells and thus reduce the recurrence risk.

Morgante et al (1999)[18] reported that patients treated with low-dose of danazol (100 mg/day for 6 months) after a laparoscopic surgery and 6 months of Gn-RH agonists therapy reduced the incidence of pelvic pain when compared with those receiving no therapy at all. Specifically, 24 months after surgery, 14 patients who were randomized to receive danazol treatment had significantly lower pain score than the other 14 patients who did not received any treatment, and the rate of recurrence, which was not clearly defined, was reported to be 44% in the former group and 67% in the latter group.

Postoperative treatment with goserelin significantly prolongs the pain-free interval after conservative surgery for symptomatic endometriosis and did not influence reproductive prognosis. It is unclear as to whether the result, which was based on as treated patients, would be any different if based on intent-to-treat patients.[19]

If women with moderate or severe dysmenorrhea given levonorgestrel-releasing intrauterine device (LNG-IUD) with the expectant management for symptomatic endometriosis following surgery, they showed a statistically significant reduction in the recurrence of dysmenorrhea 1 year after surgery in the LNG-IUD group when compared with the control group receiving a expectant management. Postoperative use of LNG-IUD reduces the medium-term risk of recurrence of moderate or severe dysmenorrhea in symptomatic endometriosis.

Although most observational studies so far have failed to find any evidence for the efficacy of postoperative medication in reducing recurrence,[20] a very recent retrospective follow-up study found that postoperative use of OC significantly reduced the risk of recurrence. They reported that patients always used OC had an absolute risk reduction of recurrence by 47% when compared with non users. In addition, the reduction appeared to depend on as how long OC was used.[21]

The use of postoperative medication may simply reflect the fact that the women who uses OC it could be sicker than those who did not, or, in the case of OC use, the users might be healthier or younger than non users.

There is insufficient evidence to conclude that hormonal suppression in association with surgery for endometriosis is associated with a significant benefit with regard to any of the outcomes identified.[22]

Even if postoperation medication proves to be effective in reducing recurrence risk, it is questionable that 'all' patients would require such medication in order to reduce the risk of recurrence. It has been reported that about 9% of women with endometriosis simply do not respond to progestin treatment, which may result from progesterone receptor isoform B (PR-B) down-regulation.[23] If PR-B is silenced due to promoter methylation, as reported in endometriosis,[24] progestin treatment or OC use may be of little value since the action of progestins is mediated mostly through PR-B. Therefore, the use of postoperation medication indiscriminately may cause unnecessary side effects (and an increase in health care costs) in some patients who may intrinsically have a much lower risk than others and in others who may be simply resistant to the therapy. The identification of high-risk patients who may benefit the most from drug intervention would remain a challenge. Finally, whether a single medication represents the optimal interventional option is debatable. The recent finding that PR-B and nuclear factor-κB (NF-κB) immunoreactivity jointly constitute a biomarker for recurrence[25] suggests the possibility that perhaps a combination of drugs may be superior to a single drug in reducing the risk of recurrence, especially if PR-B is silenced due to promoter methylation.

Medical Management of Recurrent Endometriosis

Medical treatment usually with GnRHa, oral contraceptive (OCP), progestins and danazol represents a pharmacological attempt for endometriotic lesions reduction and relief of symptoms. During the past decades, it has been shown that administration of these drugs had only temporary benfits, with no possibility to radicate endometriosis. Postoperative treatment with goserelin significantly prolonged the pain free interval after conservative surgery for symptomatic endometriosis and did not influence reproductive prognosis.[26] In addition, there are expressed consideration regarding their use immediately after laparoscopy in women desiring pregnancy, in terms of delaying conception in a critical period. In women treated with GnRHa or danazol for endometriosis associated with pelvic pain, the recurrence rates were similar and associated pain symptoms usually returned after cessation of therapy.

As far as recurrence after medical treatment is concerned, it is clear that it represents persistence of the pre-existing disease despite regression of symptoms.[27] Many studies in the past found no evidence of disease during repeat laparoscopy, while ovarian function was still pharmacologically suppressed. In contrast, laparoscopic evaluation after resumption of the ovarian function showed no significant regression of endometriosis.

OCP's administration constitutes a satisfactory option as an adjuvant treatment after surgery, for pain control and reduction of recurrence frequency and severity, when on long-term use. Many mechanisms of action, such as the reduction of menses, therefore reduction of retrograde menstruation through the tubes, suppression of ovulation and inactivation of the endometriotic implants, wherever they are located, have been proposed for the OCP's. The above mentioned mechanisms may prevent implant evolution and pro-inflammatory agent production, thus decreasing endometriosis related inflammatory reaction and pain and practically contributing to the prevention of endometriomas.

According to the Cochrane reviews, there is no sufficient data supporting that pre- or postsurgical hormonal suppression for endometriosis is associated with a significant benefit with regard to eradication of endometriosis, improvement of symptoms and pregnancy rates. There may be an improvement in AFS (American Fertility Society) scores with the presurgical sue of medical treatment.

Regarding oral progestins, reports give conflicting results about their pharmacologic mode of action in endometriosis, although they still present an acceptable option for treatment of the recurrent disease. Theories involving modulation of mitosis, locally acting growth factors and anti-inflammatory and paracrine activity have been expressed so far. Progestin's most significant advantages include effectiveness on pain relief and bleeding disorders, very good tolerability and suitability for long-term use and relatively low cost.[28]

In addition, in the era of genetics, biochemistry and molecular biology achievements, new approaches of this complex disease are needed. The generally accepted knowledge of the immune system involvement in the pathogenesis of endometriosis, through the immune cells and proinflammatory molecules may lead research in the of immune-modulators in order to control and treat the disease.

It's now generally accepted that new forms of medical treatments with no influence on normal ovulation along with surgical interventions should be the aim of the modern clinical trials.

The possible benefits should be weighed in the context of the adverse effects and costs of all these therapies.

Infertility Due to Recurrent Endometriosis

Regarding the management of infertility, current guidelines recommend surgical ablation plus adhesiolysis in stages I and II.

Laparoscopic surgical approach of endometriosis is a valuable way to improve pain symptoms, but its efficacy in treating subfertility is only modest.

Recent publications support that the probability of conception is limited and decreased after multiple operation for repetitive recurrence in contrary with others who stated that reproductive outcome is comparable to that after primary surgery. Evidence from a very recent study support the former opinion. In particular, the pregnancy rates after repetitive and first line operation were 22% and 40% respectively, while the 12 and 24 months cumulative rates were 14% and 26% for each group and, 32% and 38% for each group respectively. Ratios for patients with previous diagnosis of infertility who got preganat after reoperation and primary surgery were 19% and 34% respectively, while their 12 and 24 months cumulative rates were 13% and 22% for each group and 25% and 30% for each group respectively.

Another option that may be offered to patients with recurrent disease without ovarian endometriomas when fertility is the end-point is assisted reproductive techniques.

There is no positive relation between the number of the IVF cycles and the responsiveness to ovarian hyperstimaultion and the risk of endometriosis recurrence.

Finally, individuals who desire to get pregnant, even after oopherctomy for severe recurrent endometriosis, can do so taking advantage of IVF techniques with donor oocytes. On that occasion, of course the uterus should be preserved and adenomyosis must be excluded.

Control of Recurrence of Endometriosis

Although surgery is currently the treatment of choice for managing endo-metriosis, recurrence poses a formidable challenge. To delay or to eliminate the recurrence is presently an unmet medical need in the management of endometriosis. To this end, proposals to Investigate patterns of recurrence, to develop biomarkers for recurrence and to carry out biomarker based Interven-tion have been made.

Much research is needed to better understand the patterns of recurrence and risk factors, and to develop biomarkers. One top priority is to develop biomarkers for recurrence, which may provide much needed clues to the possible mechanisms underlying recurrence and would allow the identification of patients with high recurrence risk, and permit for targeted intervention.

⮑ SUMMARY

Endometriosis is a condition which has a debilitating nature and has enormous economic burden. Therefore, it is essential now to control the recurrence of endometriosis. Several studies have shown that the completeness or not in removing endometriotic lesions also impacts on the recurrence rate.[29] Hence, there will be a need for better, less invasive and less costly surgical techniques.

Medical treatment should not be considered as a valuable solution in cases of subfertility. However, its use is necessary to control pain when preservation of fertility.

Even if recurrence originates from *de novo* growth of endometriotic lesions, possibly derived from endometrium, the finding that COX-2 overexpression in endometriotic lesions is associated with a high-risk of recurrence suggests that COX-2 positivity in the ectopic endometrium may reflect a more favorable environment for implantation and growth of new ectopic endometrium due to altered peritoneal mesothelial cells.[30]

In view of some ambiguity and uncertainty in the efficacy of postoperative medical treatment, more well-designed and executed, better statistically powered, randomized, controlled clinical trials with longer follow-up period are acutely needed. Given the rapid advances in endometriosis research in the last 5 years, the choice of medication probably may or should not be restricted to the traditional drugs.[31] Finally, the revelation of the inner secrets of recurrence might welcome from some unlikely research areas, such as the research of endometrial stem cells. Once cell surface markers for endometrial stem cells, or better yet, markers for endometriotic stem cells, can be reliably identified, then the root cause for recurrence can be detected.

⊃ REFERENCES

1. Punnonen R, Klemi P, Nikkanen V. Recurrent endometriosis. Gynecol Obstet Invest.1980;11:307-12.
2. Candiani GB, Fedele L, Bianci S. Recurrent endometriosis. In: C. Nezhat, G. Berger, F. Nezhat, V. Buttram, C.Nezhat (Eds). Endometriosis—Advanced management and surgical techniques. Springer- Verlag. 1995;159-71.
3. Murphy AA, Green WR, Bobbie D, et al. Unsuspected endometriosis documented by scanning microscope in microscopy in visually normal peritonium. Fertil Steril. 1986;46(3):522-4.
4. Nisolle-Pochet M, Casanas-Roux F, Donnez J. Histologic study of ovarian endo-metriosis after hormonal therapy. Fertil Steril. 1988;49:423–6.
5. Vignali M, Bianchi S, Candiani M, Spadaccini G, Oggioni G, Busacca M. Surgical treatment of deep endometriosis and risk of recurrence. J Minim Invasive Gynecol 2005;12:508–13.
6. Sharpe KL, Bertero MC, Muse KN, Vernon MW. Spontaneous and steroid-induced recurrence of endometriosis after suppression by a gonadotropin-releasing hormone antagonist in the rat. Am J Obstet Gynecol. 1991;164:187–94.
7. Bulletti C, DeZiegler D, Stefanetti M, Cicinelli E, Pelosi E, Flamigni C, et al. Endometriosis: absence of recurrence in patients after endometrial ablation. Hum Reprod. 2001;16:2676–9.
8. Kunz G, Beil D, Huppert P, Leyendecker G. Structural abnormalities of the uterine wall in women with endometriosis and infertility visualized by vaginal sonography and magnetic resonance imaging. Hum Reprod. 2000;15:76–82.
9. Randall GW, Gantt PA, Poe-Zeigler RL, Bergmann CA, Noel ME, Strawbridge WR, et al. Serum antiendometrial antibodies and diagnosis of endometriosis. Am J Reprod Immunol. 2007;58:374–82.
10. Insabato L, Pettinato G. Endometriosis of the bowel with lymph node involvement. A report of three cases and review of the literature. Pathol Res Pract. 1996;192: 957– 61.
11. Luisi S, Galleri L, Marini F, Ambrosini G, Brandi ML, Petraglia F. Estrogen receptor gene polymorphisms are associated with recurrence of endometriosis. Fertil Steril 2006;85:764–6.
12. Liu X, Yuan L, Shen F, Zhu Z, Jiang H, Guo SW. Patterns of and risk factors for recurrence in women with ovarian endometriomas. Obstet Gynecol. 2007;109:1411–20.
13. Stratton P, Sinaii N, Segars J, Koziol D, Wesley R, Zimmer C, et al. Return of chronic pelvic pain from endometriosis after raloxifene treatment: a randomized controlled trial. Obstet Gynecol. 2008;111:88–96.

14. Busacca M, Marana R, Caruana P, Candiani M, Muzii L, Calia C, Bianchi S. Recurrence of ovarian endometrioma after laparoscopic excision. Am J Obstet Gynecol 1999b;180:519–23.
15. Pados G, Timpanidis J, Zafrakas M, et al. Ultrasound and MRI-imaging in preoperative evaluation of two rare cases of scar endoemtriosis. Cases J. 2008;18:97-101.
16. Donnez J, Nisolle M, Squifflet J. Ureteral endometriosis: a complication of rectovaginal endometristic (adenomyotic) nodules. Fertil Steril. 2002;77:32-7.
17. Friedlander RL. The treatment of endometriosis with danazol. J Reprod Med 1973;10:197–9.
18. Morgante G, Ditto A, La Marca A, De Leo V. Low-dose danazol after combined surgical and medical therapy reduces the incidence of pelvic pain in women with moderate and severe endometriosis. Hum Reprod. 1999;14:2371–4.
19. Vercellini P, Crosignani PG, Fadini R, Radici E, Belloni C, Sismondi P. A gonadotrophin-releasing hormone agonist compared with expectant management after conservative surgery for symptomatic endometriosis. Br J Obstet Gynaecol. 1999;106: 672–7.
20. Kikuchi I, Takeuchi H, Kitade M, Shimanuki H, Kumakiri J, Kinoshita K. Recurrence rate of endometriomas following a laparoscopic cystectomy. Acta Obstet Gynecol Scand. 2006;85:1120–4.
21. Vercellini P, Somigliana E, Daguati R, Vigano P, Meroni F, Crosignani PG. Postoperative oral contraceptive exposure and risk of endometrioma recurrence. Am J Obstet Gynecol. 2008;198:504.e1–5.
22. Yap C, Furness S, Farquhar C. Pre and postoperative medical therapy for endometriosis surgery. Cochrane Database Syst Rev. 2004;CD003678.
23. Attia GR, Zeitoun K, Edwards D, Johns A, Carr BR, Bulun SE. Progesterone receptor isoform A but not B is expressed in endometriosis. J Clin Endocrinol Metab 2000;85:2897–2902.
24. Wu Y, Kajdacsy-Balla A, Strawn E, Basir Z, Halverson G, Jailwala P, et al. Transcriptional characterizations of differences between eutopic and ectopic endometrium. Endocrinology. 2006;147:232–46.
25. Shen FH, Wang YD, Lu Y, Yuan L, Liu X, Guo SW. Immunoreactivity of progesterone receptor isoform B and nuclear factor kappa-B as biomarkers for recurrence of ovarian endometriomas. Am J Obstet Gynecol. 2008;199:486.e1–486.e10.
26. Vercellini P, Crosignani PG, Fadini R, et al. A gonadotropin releasing hormone agonist compared with expectant mangament after conservative surgery for symptomatic endometriosis. BR J Obstet Gynaecol. 1999;106(7):672-7.
27. Candiana GB, Fedele L, Bianci S. Recurrent Endometirosis. In: C Nehzat, G Berger, F Nehzat, V Buttram, C Nezhat (Eds). Endometriosis—Advanced management and surgical techniques. Springer-Verlag. 1995;159-71.
28. Schweppe KW. The place of dydrogesterone in the treatment of endometriosis and adenomyosis. Maturitas. 2009.
29. Fedele L, Bianchi S, Zanconato G, Bergamini V, Berlanda N, Carmignani L. Long-term follow-up after conservative surgery for bladder endometriosis. Fertil Steril 2005;83:1729–33.
30. Nair AS, Nair HB, Lucidi RS, Kirchner AJ, Schenken RS, Tekmal RR, et al. Modeling the early endometriotic lesion: mesothelium-endometrial cell co-culture increases endometrial invasion and alters mesothelial and endometrial gene transcription. Fertil Steril. 2008;90(4):1487–95.
31. Guo SW. Emerging drugs for endometriosis. Expert Opin Emerg Drugs. 2008;13: 547–71.

Scar Endometriosis

◀ T Ramani Devi, C Archana Devi

⊃ INTRODUCTION

Endometriosis was first described by Rokitansky in 1860. But it was only in 1903 scar endometriosis (or) cutaneous endometriosis was described by Meyer. Endometriosis is the presence and proliferation of endometrium outside the uterine cavity, more commonly in the pelvis. Prevalence of extra pelvic endometriosis is in the range of 8.9 to 15% in the literature.[1] Scar endometriosis is a rare form of extra pelvic endometriosis. It accounts for 0.07 to 0.47% in the literature.[2,3] It is more common in the abdominal skin and subcutaneous tissue compared to the muscle and fascia. Endometriosis involving only the muscle and fascia are rare. Simultaneous occurrence of pelvic endometriosis along with scar endometriosis is infrequent. It is difficult to diagnose and often confused with other surgical conditions. With careful history and clinical examination, the diagnosis should not be missed.

⊃ INCIDENCE

The actual incidence is very difficult to determine because many are under diagnosed. Though the general incidence of pelvic endometriosis varies between 10 to 15% of the reproductive age group, the incidence of scar endometriosis varies between 0.03 to 0.5% . In all series, the incidence of surgically proven endometriosis was 1.6% . The incidence is after hysterotomy is about 1.08 to 2%. Studies from India showed higher incidence following hysterotomy than LSCS . (74 to 71% Vs 6 to 4%).[3,4] Frequency of endomeriosis in and around C-section scar is 0.03 to 0.8%.[20] On analysis of 445 cases, 57% were following LSCS and 11% were following hysterotomy.[5] It occurs commonly after the surgeries in the uterus and tubes. Episiotomy site scar endometriosis is more common after postpartum curettage. Pauli and Tedeschi reported 15 cases of episiotomy site scar endometriosis out of 2208 deliveries when curettage was done and no case out of 13800 deliveries when no curettage was done. Mean age of occurrence was 31.4 years.

⊃ ETIOPATHOGENESIS OF SCAR ENDOMETRIOSIS

Scar or cutaneous endometriosis show deposits of endometrial glands and stromal cells in the dermis, subcutaneous tissue, rectus muscle and sheath.

Proposed theories of endometriosis formation are:

1. Retrograde spill of endometriosis during menstruation—(Sampson's Theory)[10]
2. Blood, lymphatic and iatrogenic spread[9,11]
3. Metaplasia of pelvic mesothelial cells[33]
4. Immune system dysfunction and autoantibody formation, drop in regulatory capacity of NK cells[29]
5. Mechanical transplantation[6-8]

Probable etiology for scar endometriosis is mechanical transplantation of viable endometrial cells into the scar during surgery which subsequently proliferate and undergo metaplasia under estrogenic influence. This theory has been demonstrated by experiments in which menstrual effluent transplanted into the abdominal wall results in scar endometriosis.

Certain risk factors are identified in hysterectomy, cesarian section, early hysterotomy less than 22 weeks, heavy menstrual flow and alcohol consumption, which may be associated with scar endometriosis.[12] Cesarean section performed before the onset of labor may increase the risk of scar endometriosis.[13] The reason for increased incidence of scar endometriosis following hysterotomy has been given as early decidua has more pluripotential capababilities and can result in cellular replication producing endometriosis. A recent study concluded that the expression of metallothionein through endometrial cells and receptor binding cancer antigen through SiSo cells (RCAS1) i.e., the membrane antigens that control cytotoxic activity, might cause the scar cells in cesarian sections to persist.[32]

Histology of Endometriosis

Macroscopy: It is appears as whitish fibrous tissue with thick chocolate colored liquid areas **(Fig. 13.1)**.

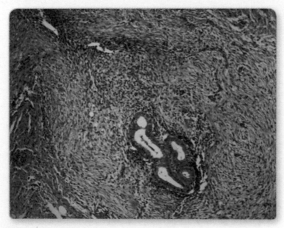

Figure 13.1: Foci of endometrial glands surrounded by myxoid stroma with an abundant presence of mesenchymal cells and siderophages (H and E × 20)

Microscopy: Major positive components of scar endometriosis are glandular and stromal elements because of hormonal influence. The glandular epithelium may have the appearance of proliferative (or) secretory (or) menstrual endometrium. Columnar, cuboidal (or) flat epithelial cells line the glands. Mitoses are frequent during the proliferative phase. Intracytoplasmic vacuoles are the hallmark of the secretory phase. Intraluminal hemorrhage and degenerative changes of epithelial cells occur in the menstural phase. Stromal components consist of a mixture of spindle cells and inflammatory cells including hemosiderin-laden macrophages. Rarely decidualization can occur.

Sites of Scar Endometriosis

Any surgery that involves contact with endometrial tissue is at-risk of scar endometriosis. Common site of scar endometriosis is in the anterior abdominal wall especially after hysterotomy, classical CS, lower segment cesarean section, hysterectomy and over the episiotomy site[15]. Anterior placenta previa is associated more with scar endometriosis **(Fig. 13.2)**.[28] Other uncommon surgeries which can also cause scar endometriosis are metroplasty, laparotomy for ectopic pregnancy and tubal ligation. It can be seen over the perineal sites following colporraphy and Bartholins' cyst excision. Rarely, it can occur following non gynecological surgeries like appendicectomy and inguinal hernia repair. After the liberal use of laparoscopic surgeries, especially for pelvic endometriosis it is seen over the umbilical and other port sites.[38] Umbilical hernias occur after laparoscopic surgery if abdominal wall fascia is not closed properly. If mesh has been used for repair in larger hernias, with concomitant inflammatory foreign body reaction it may lead to umbilical endometrioma. It is occasionally seen over the tract of amniocentesis.[39] It can also be seen over the extraperitoneal portion of round ligament in the groin. Pelviscopy is needed

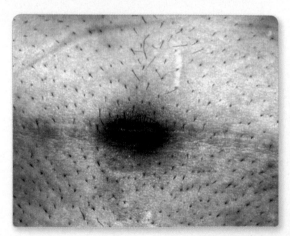

Figure 13.2: A red, tender, subcutaneous mass in the midline of the vertical cesarean scar. The overlying skin was normal

in these cases as this may be associated with intrapelvic endometriosis. One study showed 24% of patients with scar endometriosis had associated pelvic endometriosis. A case of endometriosis of the uterine wall scar following LSCS, presenting as a mass in the anterior lower part of the uterus has been reported. The time interval between the surgery and the occurrence of endometriosis may be variable, ranging between 3 months to 10 years in different series. It can happen even after 15 years. In one study by Celik et al a case was reported within 3 years of surgery. They are commonly seen within 3 to 6 years (95% CI, 2.5 to 4.8 years) after the index surgery. An incidental case of spontaneous endometriosis in a scarless abdominal wall has been reported.[21]

Clinical Presentation

Present review of 25 published cohorts from 1951 to 2006 on scar endometriosis showed classical symptoms of mass over the scar (96%), pain (87%) and 57% presented with cyclical symptoms.[5]

The usual presentation is a painful red, bluish, purple to black firm nodule in the abdominal wall in a parous women with history of gynecological or obstetrical surgery. There is often a history of delayed wound healing. The size of the nodule and the pain varies with menstrual cycle. The surface of the skin is smoother if the endometriotic nodule is deep. If the endometriosis is closer to the skin, it may present with cyclical non healing ulcers of the scar, which may show discoloration and bleeding. Very often, it is mistaken for stitch granuloma and sinuses.

Episiotomy site scar endometriosis may present as a mass over the episiotomy scar which may be tender, fixed, palpable and may extend up to the rectum.

Diagnosis of Scar Endometriosis

The diagnosis requires a detailed history taking with proper attention to the details of previous obstetric and gynecological surgeries. Presence of cyclical pain and swelling during periods are almost pathognomic.[22]

Clinical suspicion along with FNAC of the mass, USG, color Doppler, CT scan and MRI, we can reach the correct diagnosis **(Figs 13.3 and 13.4)**.[18]

USG and color Doppler can be used as a screening tool. The lesion may appear like a hypoechoic mass in the subcutaneous or fascial plane. It can be used to identify the presence of bowel loop in the mass to exclude incisional hernia with bowel obstruction.

CT scan shows a solid well-circumscribed mass but does not play any specific diagnostic role. In CT lesions appear solid, ill-defined and isodense compared with muscle and show slight enhancement. But MRI is more useful in picking up smaller masses. In endometriosis it can show iron in the hemosiderin deposits. Because of the high spatial resolution, it is better than CT scan, it can detect the planes between muscle and subcutaneous tissue and help in planning the treatment.[25,26]

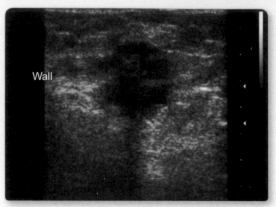

Figure 13.3: Ultrasound scan of the scar endometriosis

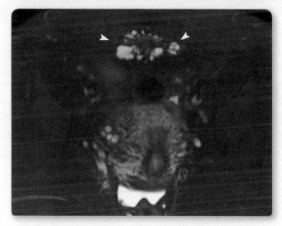

Figure 13.4: MRI of scar endometriosis

FNAC is a simple procedure that can help by giving the cytological diagnosis.[19,20,35,37] A recent report by Dwivedi et al showed that FNAC was not useful in any of the four patients who underwent this procedure. (Tru-cut biopsy may yield a better sample than FNAC).[40] However FNAC is ill-advised if an incisional hernia has to be ruled out. Smears from endometriosis show varying cellularity comprising of epithelial cells, spindle stromal cells, hemo siderin laden macrophages and inflammatory cells. Any two types of cells may give the diagnosis. Cytological features are related to cyclical hormonal changes. Histopathological diagnosis is possible only in excision biopsy.

Differential Diagnosis

Most often scar endometriosis is misdiagnosed as stitch granuloma, inguinal hernia,[34] abscess, inclusion cyst, incisional hernia, keloids, sebaceous cyst neuroma, nodular proliferative fascitis, desmoid tumor, sarcoma, lymphoma, lipoma, fat necrosis and primary metastatic cutaneous cancer especially Sister.

Mary Joseph's nodule.[23,24] There may be considerable delay in diagnosis upto 31.7 months in diagnosis and initiation of treatment.[17] This may be because most of the patients land up with general surgeons rather than gynecologist.[22]

MANAGEMENT OF SCAR ENDOMETRIOSIS

Medical Management

$NSAID_s$, danazol, progesterone, oral contraceptive pills and GnRH analogues, are used in the management of endometriosis. No medication has proved superior to other.[16] They give only partial relief of symptoms. Recently, there has been a report about the use of GnRH analogues, but they have only marginal improvement of symptoms. The size of the lesion does not change significantly. At present, there is no role for medical management of scar endometriosis. Pain reoccurs once medical management is stopped.[28]

Surgical Management

Chatterjee and Kogee reported only surgery for complete resolution of symptoms. Wide excision of the mass is the option. If there is involvement of the anterior abdominal musculature, enbloc resection of myofascial element is done. If the defect is wide then mesh can be used to close the defect.[31] Otherwise layer closure is sufficient in most of the cases. With the negative margin very rarely scar endometriosis of LSCS scar breach the pelvic peritoneum.[30] Regarding the episiotomy site scar, wide excision is needed. If it involves the anal sphincter, it has to be repaired carefully after the wide excision (Anal sphincteroplasty).[45]

Malignant Risk following Scar Endometriosis

Malignant change is very rare.[14] Longstanding recurrent scar endometriosis can undergo malignant change as adenocarcinoma, adenosarcoma, clear cell carcinoma[27] and endometroid carcinoma. Only 1% of cases of malignant transformation of endometriosis occur at extrapelvic sites and 4% over the laparotomy scars. Treatment is wide surgical excision with mesh replacement. There was a case report of malignant transformation of a large scar endometrioma.[36] The interval between the onset of scar endometriosis to malignant transformation varies from a few months to 40 years.

FOLLOW-UP AND PREVENTION OF SCAR ENDOMETRIOSIS

Follow-up is a must as scar endometriosis can reoccur, which needs repeat wide incision. In repeated reoccurrences, malignancy has to be considered. Episiotomy site scar endometriosis rarely reoccurs—reoccurrence rate 4.3%.

Good surgical technique with proper care during surgeries involving uterus, tubes and ovaries may help to prevent scar endometriosis. Lifting the uterus outside of the pelvis before making the uterine incision was shown to significantly reduce the likelihood of developing abdominal wall endometriosis.[3,41] Other ideas include using separate needles for the uterine and abdominal closure,[3] removing a functional corpus luteum at the time of a hysterectomy,[3] using high-pressure irrigation,[42] not using a sponge to clean the endometrial cavity, and prophylactic hormonal therapy after hysterectomy.[43,44] Although these techniques may seem intuitively pleasing, none has been tested rigorously. If hysterotomy is done before 22 weeks, there is increased chances of scar endometriosis.[12] Fortunately, now the incidence of hysterotomies have come down and replaced by medical termination. With the increase in the incidence of laparoscopic surgeries, endometriosis of the port sites can be avoided by retrieving the specimens in endobags which will avoid the direct contact with the port sites.

Author's Personal Experience with Scar Endometriosis

In the author's experience all the cases were clinically diagnosed as scar endometriosis except one which was thought to be a foreign body granuloma. No case had preoperative FNAC. These patients were subjected to USG to rule out intraperitoneal endometriosis. MRI has the advantage of being more accurate regarding the diagnosis and its location. This made the author do MRI only in the recent cases. All these cases were managed only by the gynecologist and mesh was not used in any of these cases. HPE confirmed the diagnosis in all cases. Postoperative follow-up showed no recurrences till date.

I have had 8 cases of scar endometriosis during the past 10 years. 4 cases following LSCS, 1 case after hysterotomy and LSCS, 1 case after laparoscopy, and 2 cases at the episiotomy site.

Case 1

G2 P1 L1, previous LSCS, LCB 4 years came with history of 3 months amenorrhea and swelling in the right side of the previous pfannensteil scar for the past 6 months. Skin over the scar was normal. The mass was around 3 to 4 cm and tender. The mass increased in size during menstruation. Hence, a clinical diagnosis of scar endometriosis was made. Since she was planned for elective LSCS, wide excision was done during the subsequent surgery. HPE proved to be scar endometriosis.

Case 2 and 3

Both were similar cases, who reported with the swelling over the previous scars, which enlarged during periods. The swelling was in the abdominal wall over the previous pfannensteil scar. The duration between the onset of masses in both cases were around 4 to 5 years. Both had wide excision of the masses. There were no reoccurrence for the past 3 years. One patient had a pregnancy following excision and repeat surgery showed no evidence of scar endometriosis.

Case 4

A 36 years old lady with previous hysterotomy for premarital pregnancy and then a LSCS done around 6 years ago, came with a swelling over the scar for the past 3 years. The patient had severe dysmenorrhea and painful enlargement of the scar during periods. USG was done, which showed adenomyosis of uterus around 14 weeks and a hypoechoic mass around 4 cm in the subcutaneous plane, which was diagnosed as scar endometriosis. The patient was posted for abdominal hysterectomy along with excision of the scar endometriosis. Patient became asymptomatic after the surgery.

Case 5 and 6

Both patients were para 1, had normal vaginal deliveries and last child birth between 3 to 4 years, came with complaints of painful swelling over the episiotomy scar during periods. One patient had the swelling over the middle of the episiotomy scar. Other one had swelling near the fourchette and was having dyspareunia and dyschezia. Clinically first patient had a defined mass over the middle of right episiotomy scar around 2 × 2 cm. Rectum and vagina were free. She underwent wide excision and was fine. Second patient had endometriosis involving the right lateral wall of the rectum, which could be felt during the rectal examination. Hence, the need for rectal resection and colostomy if needed was explained to the patient. She underwent wide excision of the scar up to the rectum. Right lateral wall of rectum was opened and the endometriotic areas excised. Rectum was closed in 2 layers and layer closure of the perineum was done. Postoperative period was uneventful.

Case 7

This was a girl of 16 years who had laparoscopic excision of non communicating horn of the left side. She had left ovarian endometrioma also. Endometrioma was excised along with the left horn and removed through a mini incision in the left lateral port. Patient came back 3 years later with a swelling over the mini lap scar. MRI was done. This showed a mass in the subcutaneous plane, and other horn of the uterus was normal. She underwent excision of the scar, which proved to be scar endometriosis. This was the youngest patient with scar endometriosis the author had and literature search did not reveal any patient younger than this. Minimum age described was 18 years in one study.[5]

Case 8

A lady with previous 2 LSCS done through RPM scar came with recurrent non healing ulcers and sinuses over the scar since the last surgery which was done around 2 years ago. Clinical diagnosis of foreign body granuloma was thought and the patient underwent wide excision of the scar. The HPE was reported as scar endometriosis. This was the only case where clinical diagnosis was missed.

⊃ CONCLUSION

Scar endometriosis though very rare and affect females between 20 to 40 years continues to be a diagnostic challenge. The incidence of cesarean section, hysterectomies, laparoscopic surgeries, amniocentesis are on the increase. So the chances of scar endometriosis are also going to be high. Hence, it is of utmost importance to modify the practices at the time of surgery, to prevent the deposition of endometrial tissues over the scar. Increased awareness and high index of suspicion along with high-tech diagnostic modalities will clinch the diagnosis and guide towards proper management. Medical management is unsuccessful, therefore surgery should be offered to these patients and it is usually successful. These women need follow-up also.

⊃ REFERENCES

1. Bergqvist A. Different types of extragenital endometriosis: a review. Gynaecol Endocrinol. 1993;7:207-21.
2. Wolf GC, Singh KB. Caesarean scar endometriosis: a review. Obstet Gynaecol Surv. 1989;44:89-95.
3. Chatterjee SK. Scar endometriosis: a clinicopathologic study of 17 cases. Obstet Gynaecol. 1980;56:81–4.
4. Rani PR, Soundararaghavan S, Rajaram P. Endometriosis in abdominal scars—review of 27 cases. Int J Gynaecol Obstet.1991;36:215–18
5. Horton J D, Dezee K J, Ahnfeldt E P, Wagner M..Abdominal wall endometriosis: A Surgeon's perspective and review of 445 cases. Am J Surg 2008;196(2) 207-12.
6. Francica G. Abdominal wall endometriosis near caesarean delivery scars-sonographic and color Doppler findings in a series of 12 patients. J Ultrasound Med 2003;22:1041-7.
7. Kaloo P, Reid G, Wong F. Caesarean section scar endometriosis: Two cases of recurrent diseases and literature review.
8. Tanos B, Anteby SO. Caesarean section scar endometriosis. Int J Gynaecol Obstet 1994:47: 163-66
9. Higgins JP, Thompson SG, Deeks JJ, et al. Measuring inconsistency in meta-analyses. BMJ. 2003;327:557–560.
10. Luciano AA, Pitkin RM. Endometriosis: approaches to diagnosis and treatment. Surg Annu. 1984;16:297–312.
11. Halban J.Metastatic hystroadenosis.Wien Klin Wichenschr 1924;37:1205-6.
12. De oliveira MA, de leon AC, Friere EC, de Oliveira HC. Risk Factors for abdominal scar endometriosis after obstetric hysterotomies. A case control study. Acta Obstet Gynecol Scand 2007 ; 86(1) : 73-80.
13. Wicherek L, Klimek M, Skret M, et al. The obstetrical history in patients with Pfannenstiel scar endometriosis- an analysis of 81 patients. Gynecol Obstet Invest, 2007; 63(2):107-13
14. Leng J, Lang J, Guo L, Li H, Liu Z. Carcinosarcoma arising from atypical endometriosis in a cesarean section scar. Int. J Gynecol Cancer 2006 ; 16 ; 432-35
15. Teng CC,Yang HM,Chen KF, et al. Abdominal wall endometriosis: an over looked possibly preventable complication. Yaiwan J Obstet Gynecol 2008 47 (1) : 42-8.
16. Ozlean S, Arici A. Advances in treatment options of endometriosis. Gynaecol Obstet Invest 2009 ; 67 : 81-91.
17. Agarwal A, Fong YF. Cutaneous endometriosis. Singapore Med J. 2008;49(9):704-9.

18. Pados G, Tympanidis J, Zafrakers M, et al. Ultrasound MR Imaging in preoperative evaluation of two rare cases of scar endometriosis. Cases Journal 2008 1(1):97.
19. Gupta RK. Fine needle aspiration cytodiagnosis of endometriosis in C Section scar and rectus sheath mass lesions—a study of seven cases. Diag Cyto Pathol 2008,36 (4):224-6.
20. Lamblin G, Mathevert P, Buenerd A. Parietal endometriosis in abdominal scars. Report of 3 cases. J Gynecol Obstet Bio Reprod 1999;28:271-4.
21. Ideyi SC, Schein M, Niazi M, Gerst PH. Spontaneous endometriosis of the abdominal wall . Dig Sur 2003; 20:246-48.
22. Singh KK, Lessels AM, Adam DJ, et al. Presentation of endometriosis to general surgeons: a 10 year experience. Br J Surg 1995;82:1349-51.
23. Woodward PJ, Sohaey R, Mezzetti TP. Endometriosis; radiologic- pathologic correlation. Radiographics 2001;21:193-216
24. Wolf C, Obrist P, Ensinger C Sonographic features of abdominal wall endometriosis. AJR 1997;169:916-17.
25. Coley BD, Casola G. Incisional endometrioma involving the rectus abdominis muscle and subcutaneous tissues: CT appearance . AJR 1993;160:549-50
26. Wolf GC, Kopecky KK. MR imaging of endometriosis arising in cesarean section scar. J comput Assist Tomogr 1989;13:150-52
27. Miller DM, Schouls JJ, Ehlen TG. Clear cell carcinoma arising in extragonadal endometriosis in a caesarean section scar during pregnancy. Gynecol Oncol. 1998 70;127-130.
28. Schoelefield HJ, Sajjad Y, Morgan PR. Cutaneous endometriosis and its association with caesarean section and gynaecological procedures. J obstet Gynaecol 2002;22:553-2.
29. Hernandez Valencia M, Zarate A, Hernandez Quijano T. Endometriosis in delayed scarring of postpartum eutocis episiorrhaphy integral aspect and a case report. Rev Med Inst Mex Seguro Soc. 2005;43:237-42.
30. Philip K, Reid G, Wong F. Caesarean section scar endometriosis: two cases of recurrent disease and a literature review. Aust NZ J Obstet Gynaecol. 2002;42(2):218–20.
31. Khetan N, Torkington J, Watkin A, et al. Endometriosis: presentation to general surgeons. Ann R Coll Surg Eng I. 1999;81:255-9.
32. Wicherek L, Dutsch-Wicherek M, Galazka K, et al. Comparison of RCAS1 and metallothianein expression and the presence and activity of immune cells in human ovarian and abdominal wall endometriomas. Reprod Biol Endocrinol. 2006;4:41.
33. Steck WD, Helwig EB. Cutaneous endometriosis. Clin Obstet Gynecol. 1966;9:373–83.
34. Clausen I, Nielsen KT. Endometriosis in the groin. Int J Gynaecol Obstet. 1987;25: 469–71.
35. Hensen JH, Van Breda Vriesman AC, Puylaert JB. Abdominal wall endometriosis: clinical presentation and imaging features with emphasis on sonography. AJR Am J Roentgenol. 2006;186:616–20.
36. Madsen H, Hansen P, Andersen OP. Endometrioid carcinoma in an operation scar. Acta Obstet Gynecol Scand. 1980;59:475–6.
37. Simsir A, Thorner K, Waisman J, et al. Endometriosis In abdominal scars: a report of three cases diagnosed by fine-needle aspiration biopsy. Am Surg. 2001;67:984–6.
38. Sirito R, Puppo A, Centurioni MG, et al. Incisional hernia on the 5-mm trocar port site and subsequent wall endometriosis on the same site: a case report. Am J Obstet Gynecol. 2005;193:878–80.
39. Kaunitz A, Di Sant' Agnese PA. Needle tract endometriosis: an unusual complication of amniocentesis. Obstet Gynecol. 1979;54:753-5.

40. Dwivedi AJ, Agarwal SN, Silva YJ. Abdominal wall endometriomas. Dig Dis Sci 2002;22:553-4.
41. Martin RH, Higginbottom J. Hysterotomy and endometriosis. Lancet. 1973;2:106.
42. Wasfie T, Gomez E, Seon S, et al. Abdominal wall endometrioma after cesarean section; a preventable complication. Int Surg. 2002;87:175-7.
43. Tanos V, Anteby SO. Cesarean scar endometriosis. Int J Gynaecol Obstet. 1994; 47:163-6.
44. Koger KE, Shatney CH, Hodge K, et al. Surgical scar endometrioma. Surg Gynecol Obstet. 1993;177:243-6.
45. Barisic GI, Krivokapic ZV, Jonanovic DR. Perineal endometriosis in episiotomy scar with anal sphincter involvement: report of two cases review of the literature. Int Urogynecol J Pelvic Floor Dysfunct. 2006;17(6):646-9.

Rectovaginal Endometriosis: A Distinct Entity

◀ Madhavi Panpalia, Neeta Warty, Firuza Rajesh Parikh

➲ INTRODUCTION

Endometriosis is the most frequent cause of pelvic pain in women of reproductive age and may cause prolonged suffering and disability, negatively affecting health-related quality of life.[1]

➲ DEFINITION

Deep invasive endometriosis involves the Douglas pouch, the rectovaginal septum, intestine, anterior pouch and the uterosacral ligaments.[2]

Its characteristics are unique and so they should be considered as a distinct entity. There is a difference in lesion characteristics, histology, clinical parameters and therapeutic response.

Rectovaginal endometriosis (RVE), which is the most important type of deep endometriosis, consists of endometriotic nodules, in which the fibrotic component is prevalent, within the connective tissue between the anterior rectal wall and the vagina.[3] The lesions often reorganize the pelvic anatomy by dense fibrotic adhesions that cover the deep lesions and cause contraction of the rectovaginal pouch, involving the rectosigmoid.[3] It often infiltrates the posterior vaginal and anterior rectal walls[4] which usually causes symptoms such as disabling dysmenorrhea, deep dyspareunia limiting sexual activity, chronic pelvic pain and severe dyschezia and impaired quality of life. It is a chronic disease with a high-risk of pain recurrence.[5] In fact, women with this form of the disease have significant risks of both bowel and urinary tract involvement. Such significant levels of pathology makes surgery very complex and requires expertise, with better outcomes obtained in specialized centers.[3]

➲ INCIDENCE

Rectovaginal septum endometriosis occurs infrequently.[6] RVE causing obliteration of the cul-de-sac accounts for 5 to 10% of cases of endometriosis **(Fig. 14.1)**.[7]

Etiology

Endometriosis remains an enigmatic disease, which is problematic because the pathogenesis is still uncertain and the incidence of recurrence is high. The etiology of RVE is still a matter of debate.

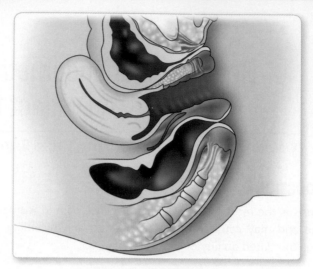

Figure 14.1: Location of RVE

Two theories have been implicated.

Retrograde menstruation Sampon's theory: There is retrograde flow of menstrual blood through the uterine tubes during menstruation. The endometrial fragments get implanted in the peritoneal surface of the pelvic organs (dependent sites). Subsequently, cyclic growth and shedding of the endometrium at the ectopic sites occur under the influence of endogenous ovarian hormones.

Coelomic metaplasia Meyer and Ivanoff theory: Chronic irritation of the pelvic peritoneum by the menstrual blood may cause coelomic metaplasia which results in endometriosis. Alternatively, the Mullerian tissue remnants maybe trapped within the peritoneum. They could undergo metaplasia and be transformed into endometrium.

Symptoms

RVE is strongly associated with pelvic pain (non-menstrual), painful menstruation (dysmenorrhea), pain during defecation (dyschezia), deep dyspareunia, and poor quality of life.

The type of endometriosis is not related to the frequency and severity of dysmenorrhea and non-menstrual pain. There is no clear-cut association between stage, site or morphological characteristics of pelvic endometriosis and pain.[8]

When rectal infiltration occurs, dyschezia and rectal bleeding can be observed.[9]

Staging

At laparoscopy, patients are staged according to the American Fertility Society (AFS).

RVE is graded according to the Adamyan system.[3] Briefly, the condition is considered to be:

1. Stage 1 when the endometriotic lesion is confined in the rectovaginal tissue.
2. Stage 2 when the vaginal wall is invaded with lesions visible at the posterior fornix.
3. Stage 3 when the lesion spreads into the sacrouterine ligaments and rectal serosa.
4. Stage 4 when the rectal wall, rectosigmoid zone, and rectouterine peritoneum are completely involved.

⊃ DIAGNOSIS

RVE is difficult to assess by clinical examination and infiltration of the rectal wall can only be suspected in 40 to 68% of the cases.[4] It is assessed before intervention by means of pelvic and rectal examination usually performed at the time of menstruation.[3] Even during laparoscopy, gynecologists may fail to diagnose RVE or fail to estimate the extension of an endometriotic lesion in the rectovaginal septum. Therefore, imaging techniques are mandatory during the preoperative work-up. Preoperative evaluation is mandatory for the selection of different medical or surgical options.[2] Diagnosis is confirmed at surgery and ultimately by histologic evidence of endometrial-like glands and stroma surrounded by fibrosis and smooth muscle hyperplasia in the rectovaginal septum.[3]

Physical Examination

It may not be very accurate. Examination of the patient may show the following:
* Visualization of lesions on the posterior vaginal fornix
* Infiltration or a nodule involving the pouch of Douglas on vaginal examination
* Infiltration or a mass involving the rectosigmoid colon on rectal digital examination.

Obtaining a diagnostic image of RVE, the most severe, advanced stage of endometriosis, is difficult. Transabdominal ultrasonography, transvaginal ultrasonography, rectosigmoidoscopy, as well as computerized tomography and nuclear magnetic resonance, may not accurately assess the extension of endometriosis into the rectovaginal septum.[6] In addition, several imaging methods have been used in the attempt to improve the noninvasive diagnosis of rectal infiltration in women with RVE. Different studies have been conducted using modified imaging techniques to improve the detection rate of RVE.

Transvaginal Ultrasonography

Transvaginal sonography (TVS) should be considered the first-line procedure.[2,10] It can detect endometriotic foci, but its sensitivity is poor for the diagnosis and workup of posterior pelvic lesions.[6] It is not a reliable method in the assessment of RVE. In TVS, the operator obtains longitudinal and transversal scans of the uterus, and particular attention is given to the rectovaginal septum for the detection of endometriotic lesions.[6] The rectovaginal septum is considered to be involved when a nodule or mass is found below the horizontal plane passing through the lower border of the posterior lip of the cervix (under the peritoneum).[11] The vagina is considered to be involved when the posterior vaginal fornix is thickened, with or without a round cystic anechoic area. The rectum/sigmoid colon is considered to be involved when an irregular hypoechoic mass is found, with or without hypoechoic or hyperechoic foci, penetrating into the intestinal wall.[11]

Transvaginal Tenderness Guided Ultrasonography[2]

Some modifications have been made in the regular TVS for improving the accuracy of identifying deep endometriosis. Transvaginal tenderness-guided ultrasonography is performed by using an acoustic window between the transvaginal probe and the surrounding vaginal structures by increasing the amount of ultrasound gel inside the probe cover. In addition, because the endometriotic nodule itself can induce pain, patients are asked to indicate during the ultrasonographic examination which points feel tender under gentle pressure of the probe, and particular attention is paid to evaluate these sites. This approach has high sensitivity and specificity.

Deep endometriosis implants are suspected from the presence of hypoechoic linear thickening or nodules/masses with or without regular contours in five locations:

i. Vaginal walls
ii. Rectovaginal septum
iii. Rectosigmoid involvement
iv. Uterosacral ligaments
v. Anterior compartment (anterior pouch and/or bladder).

In particular, rectosigmoid involvement is suspected in cases which show the presence of nodules which have thin band-like echoes departing from the center of the mass that are defined as 'Indian head dress' **(Figs 14.2 and 14.3)**. Also the anterior compartment is examined to evaluate the presence of bladder endometriosis. Transvaginal ultrasonography combined with water-contrast in the rectum.

RWC-TVS

Another modification in the traditional TVS is when it is combined with a water contrast in the rectum.[12] The latter is distended by injecting saline solution and a TVS performed. RVE appears as rounded or triangular hypoechoic masses, located anterior or lateral to the rectum, immediately adjacent or close to the rectal wall **(Figs 14.4 and 14.5)**.[4] Rectal infiltration is diagnosed when a rectovaginal hypoechoic mass penetrates into the intestinal wall thickening the muscularis mucosa.[12] Although there is a trend for RWC-TVS to have higher accuracy than TVS in diagnosing RVE, the difference between the two techniques was not found to be statistically significant in the initial study by Menada et al.[4] Moreover, RWC-TVS is unsuitable for diagnosing endometriotic nodules located above the rectosigmoid junction which are beyond the field of view of ultrasonography.[4] RWC-TVS is more accurate than TVS in diagnosing rectal infiltration reaching at least the muscularis propria in women with RVE.[4] However, this exam cannot determine whether the infiltration reaches the rectal submucosa. RWC-TVS may be more painful than TVS, therefore it could be used when TVS cannot exclude the presence of rectal infiltration in women with RVE.[4]

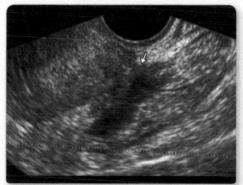

Figure 14.2: Transvaginal sonography—Indian head dress sign in rectal involvement (*Courtesy*: Dr CP Lulla)

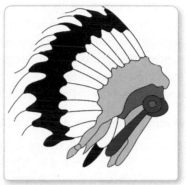

Figure 14.3: Indian head dress

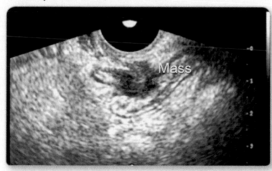

Figure 14.4: B mode which shows Hypoechoic mass lesion with speculated margins and rectal involvement in rectovaginal endometriosis (*Courtesy*: Dr CP Lulla)

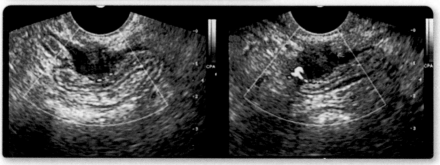

Figure 14.5: Same lesion on color Doppler shows increased vascularity in the endometriotic lesion in the rectovaginal septum (*Courtesy*: Dr CP Lulla)

Rectal Endoscopic Ultrasonography (RES)

Several studies have reported the effectiveness of RES in the diagnosis of deep pelvic endometriosis, and in particular of RVE, with a high sensitivity and specificity. Deep pelvic endometriosis is defined by the presence of a hypoechoic nodule or mass, with or without regular contours in the rectovaginal septum.[11] The largest diameter of the lesions, their location relative to the anal margins and infiltration of adjacent pelvic organs can be assessed. In the rectum and/or sigmoid colon, involvement of the muscularis propria (hypoechoic and thin) can be distinguished from the hyperechoic submucosa and mucosa.[13]

After a simple rectal enema, an echo endoscope operating at 7.5 and 12 Hz is positioned in the sigmoid and then slowly withdrawn through the sigmoid and rectum. Studies of the bowel wall and adjacent areas can be carried out by moving the probe up and down several times before and after instilling water into the intestinal lumen.[13] The procedure can be performed under general anesthesia, or with local or topical anesthesia.

Magnetic Resonance Imaging (MRI)

Deep pelvic endometriosis is defined as subperitoneal infiltration of endo-metrial tissue. These are typically found in the rectum and rectovaginal septum, though other fibromuscular structures like uterosacral ligaments, vagina, or bladder may also be involved **(Fig. 14.6)**. Infiltrating lesions of the posterior cul-de-sac are either intraperitoneal or retroperitoneal in location. Endometriotic implants trigger an inflammatory response in the dependent portion of the pouch of Douglas, resulting in adhesions between the surfaces of the anterior rectal wall and posterior vaginal fornix, with subsequent wall infiltration. These retroperitoneal posterior cul-de-sac lesions are subclassified into groups as defined with transrectal ultrasonography and MR imaging: rectovaginal septum lesions (type I), posterior wall forniceal lesions (type II), and hourglass-shaped lesions (type III). Rectovaginal septum lesions are usually

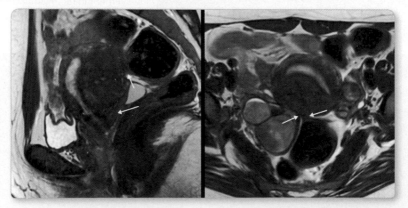

Figure 14.6: MRI. Rectouterine adhesions due to serosal endometrial deposits
(*Courtesy*: Dr Karthik Ganesan)

small implants located between the posterior vaginal wall and the anterior rectal wall, not attached to the cervix, and account for approximately 10% of cases. Posterior forniceal lesions are located between from the posterior fornix and the rectovaginal septum, without extension to the rectal wall, and account for 65% of cases. Hourglass-shaped lesions are larger lesions, which represent extension of the posterior forniceal lesions to the anterior rectal wall and are seen in 25% of cases.

On MR imaging, deep endometriotic implants appear dark to intermediate in signal intensity with punctate regions of high T1 signal intensity, and uniform dark in signal intensity on T2-weighted images, with profuse and delayed enhancement due to the coexisting inflammatory fibrosis. Additionally diffuse or focal thickening of the rectal wall, with or without posterosuperior retraction of the posterior fornix may also be identified. Depiction of deep rectal involvement with MR imaging is difficult with approximate sensitivity of 33%. Improved results are noted with the use of phased-array coils, endovaginal coils, and rectal enema.[14]

Sonovaginography[6]

Sonovaginography is a new technique, for the assessment of RVE which consists of TVS combined with the introduction of saline solution to the vagina. Each patient is asked to partially empty her bladder, thus leaving a small amount of urine within to enhance visualization of the anterior vaginal wall and of the vesicovaginal septum during the procedure. The solution, once in the vaginal channel, creates an acoustic window between the transvaginal probe and the surrounding structures of the vaginal channel. Moreover, the saline solution exerts a pressure in the vaginal channel that distends the vaginal walls, permitting enhanced visualization of the vaginal walls, vaginal fornix, uterosacral ligaments, pouch of Douglas, rectovaginal septum, and vesicovaginal septum. With this technique, endometriotic lesions can be detected as hypoechoic, irregular lesions at the level of the vaginal wall; the lesions are most often found infiltrating the surrounding structures and the uterosacral ligaments. Once an endometriotic lesion is detected, its location, size, extension, and infiltration are evaluated. It is a reliable method for the assessment of RVE: it is simple in its performance and provides information on location, extension, and infiltration of endometriotic lesions in the rectovaginal septum, which are important in selecting the kind of surgery to be performed. These preliminary results strongly encourage the use of this technique in the assessment of RVE but because of the small number of patients included in the studies, further studies are necessary.

Introital Three-dimensional (3D) Transvaginal Sonography (US)[10]

In introital 3D-US examinations are performed with the transducer placed on the perineum. The transducer is placed quite firmly against the symphysis pubis without causing significant discomfort. To acquire a correct volume, the symphysis pubis, urethra, vagina, and rectum should be visualized in the same image. Introital 3D-US seems to be an effective means of detecting endometriosis of the rectovaginal septum and should be included in preoperative evaluation in patients with clinical suspicion of RVE.

3D-US has at least three advantages over the traditional 2D-US:
1. It seems to be highly reproducible, and the image can be reconstructed after a single sweep of the ultrasound beam across the target—may be very useful to correctly locate the lesions in the pelvis evaluating the spatial relationship with other organs.
2. It may allow unrestricted access to an infinite number of viewing planes—may allow an evaluation even after the first acquisition to further study the involvement of the ureter or the bowel.
3. Stored 3D volumes can be reassessed and compared by the same or different examiners over time—may be relevant for monitoring the effect of medical therapies over a period of time.

However, further studies in a larger population will be necessary to confirm its role.

Colonoscopy

It is inaccurate in the diagnosis of bowel endometriosis because endometriotic lesions predominantly affect the serosa, muscularis and submucosa.[4]

Multislice Computed Tomography Enteroclysis (MSCTe)[4]

Multislice computerized tomography combined with retrograde distension of the colon by rectal enteroclysis (MSCTe) has been proved to be effective in the diagnosis of bowel endometriosis. This technique reliably identifies endometriotic nodules located on the sigmoid colon, cecum and ileum; however, some rectal nodules may be missed by MSCTe.[4] Subsequently, it was found to have similar accuracy in the diagnosis of rectosigmoid endometriosis when compared with RWC-TVS. It may be effective in determining the presence and depth of bowel involvement, however further studies are warranted.

Rectal Involvement

Various imaging modalities have been used to detect rectal involvement in RVE, particularly the MRI and RES. Various studies have been done comparing the effectiveness of one over the other. Some studies have found both equally accurate in detecting rectal involvement[13] while others have found RES to be more better in the diagnosis of rectal involvement.[15] Prospective studies with a large number of patients are needed in order to validate the results.

Surgically

RVE is recognized as cul-de-sac obliteration (CDSO) at the time of surgery.[16] The presence or type of CDSO is determined according to the American Society for Reproductive Medicine Classification, that is, the cul-de-sac is diagnosed as normal when the bulge of the posterior vaginal vault is between both uterosacral ligaments. As partial cul-de-sac obliteration (PCDSO) when only part of the bulge of the posterior fornix is seen, and as complete cul-de-sac obliteration (CCDSO) when the posterior vaginal vault cannot be seen at all.[16]

⊃ HISTOLOGY

Histologically, RVE is considered a specific entity of deep endometriosis, when endometriotic cells have infiltrated the peritoneum at least 5 mm below the surface.[17] The histological criteria used for the diagnosis of pelvic endometriosis included the presence of ectopic endometrial tissue (ectopic glands together with stroma). It is surrounded by fibrosis and smooth muscle hyperplasia in the rectovaginal septum.[3]

The rectovaginal lesion may extend to the superficial muscularis or deeper up to the mucosa of the rectum or vagina. In the coronal plane this lesion extends laterally and may merge with the uterosacral lesion. When this occurs bilaterally there is true cul-de-sac obliteration by a continuous sheet of fibrotic endometriosis.

⊃ TREATMENT

RVE usually causes distressing pain. Pain associated with endometriosis may be treated with surgery or drugs. Surgical treatment may be effective but is associated with a high-risk of morbidity and major complications. Information on the effect of medical alternatives for pain relief in this condition is scarce.[1]

Because endometriosis is a benign disease, and since in a large number of cases there is no definitive best therapeutic solution, the choice between the available treatment alternatives should be shared with the patient.[18]

The management of deeply infiltrating endometriosis should be to improve the woman's quality of life and addressing fertility issues when relevant.[3]

Along this line, the Practice Committee of the American Society for Reproductive Medicine (2008) has recently stated that 'endometriosis should be viewed as a chronic disease that requires a life-long management plan with the goal of maximizing the use of medical treatment and avoiding repeated surgical procedures'.[1]

The currently used staging system of the disease has little prognostic value when it comes to predicting the risk of recurrence.[3]

Medical

Current practice erroneously takes for granted that medical treatments are not effective for RVE.[7] Endometriosis of the rectovaginal septum is uncommon, and there is no known and accepted medical treatment.[19] Only few investigators have studied medical treatment aimed specifically at endometriosis of the rectovaginal septum.[19]

An important role of estrogens in the pathogenesis of endometriosis is widely accepted to date. Medical treatments for endometriosis have focused on the hormonal alteration of the menstrual cycle in an attempt to produce a state of pseudopregnancy, pseudomenopause, or chronic anovulation.

Good results are also obtainable with drugs for these patients, provided bowel and ureteral stenosis or adnexal masses with doubtful characteristics are ruled out.[1] The best candidates for long-term medical treatment are subjects not wanting pregnancy, those who have undergone unsuccessful operation, women who have already undergone nonradical interventions who might prefer to avoid further surgery, women who may want to postpone reoperation or do not accept the risk of additional morbidity.[20] Non-responders, non-compliants, and those who are unwilling to take medications for years even if well-tolerated, should consider surgery.[1] Medical treatment in women with RVE is effective in terms of pain relief, lesion reduction during therapy, improvement in health related-quality of life, and patient satisfaction.[1] Symptomatic endometriosis is suppressed but not cured by hormonal therapies, and pain recurrence is frequent after the withdrawal of drugs.[21] Measurement of pain variation for assessment during the different study period was by means of visual analogue (VAS) or verbal rating (VRS) scales.[1] Patient was asked to complete a questionaire on the presence and severity of dysmenorrhea, nonmenstrual pelvic pain, and deep dyspareunia.

Medical treatment should be continued for long periods. Primary end point is degree of patient satisfaction with treatment.[21]

In light of the considerable likelihood of postoperative pain and lesion recurrence gynecologists and patients should be aware that the real choice may not reveal to be between medical treatment and surgery, but instead between medical treatment alone and surgery followed by prolonged pharmacological therapy. However, only the results of an adequately designed randomized trial on hormonal therapy versus excision could definitively disentangle this issue.[1]

Finally, it should be remembered that, although RVE is a benign condition with limited tendency to progress, periodic evaluation to exclude silent obstructive uropathy should be systematically scheduled.[1]

Specific considerations on individual drugs should take into account not only antalgic efficacy, but also safety, tolerability and cost. As an example, Gn-RH agonists appear unsuitable for long-term treatments when used alone, due to severe metabolic and subjective side effects. Combination with 'add-back' therapies may alleviate untoward consequences, but further increases the already high cost of this class of drugs.[1]

The development of new drugs and alternative routes of administration is the object of several research efforts, as well as the attempts to prolong the beneficial effects of these agents.[22]

Progestogens and Estrogen-Progestogen

Progestogens and estrogen-progestogen combinations have been repeatedly demonstrated to be safe, well-tolerated, inexpensive and effective in the long-term treatment of women with symptomatic endometriosis.[20,21] It reduces the symptoms of dysmenorrhea, dyspareunia and dyschezia.[20] Prolonged medical treatment with progestogen and estrogen-progestogen combinations has been demonstrated to successfully suppress ectopic implants, relieve pain symptoms, and improve health-related quality of life thus offering a valuable alternative to serial surgery.[21] Unfortunately, very few data published on its efficacy in RVE.[20]

Progestogens

Progestogens have been demonstrated to be safe, well-tolerated, inexpensive and effective in the long-term treatment of women. Unfortunately, data on the efficacy of progestogens in women with RVE are limited.[20] Progestogen treatments are symptomatic and do not cure deep-infiltrating disease.[20]

Norethisterone acetate: It is a strong progestin derivative of 19-nortestosterone which offers various advantages in relieving pelvic pain for the long-term treatment of endometriosis. It allows good control of uterine bleeding as compared with other compounds, has a positive effect on calcium metabolism by producing greater increases in bone mineral density, and at low dosages has limited effects on the lipoprotein profile.[1] They are associated with weight gain and androgenic side-effects.[20]

It reduces the symptoms of dysmenorrhea, dyspareunia and dyschezia.[20]

The use of progestins for symptomatic RVE is further supported by biological evidence on the essential role of mast cells in promoting inflammation.[1] Progesterone inhibits mast cell secretion and reduces production of prostaglandins and cytokines which stimulate pain fibers.[20]

It has been used successfully as "add-back" therapy in combination with long-term GnRH agonist treatment for symptomatic endometriosis however some studies show similar results using norethindrone acetate alone in symptomatic endometriosis.

Cyproterone acetate: This progestogen was tried as an alternative to traditional norethindrone acetate in a study by Vercellini et al in 2005. It is a 17-hydroxyprogesterone derivative with antiandrogenic and antigonadotropic properties, which has been used successfully orally in treatment of RVE.[20] It is usually very well-tolerated and it generally achieves good uterine bleeding control.[20] Low dose of ethinyl estradiolare added in order to limit estrogen-deprivation effects without stimulating endometriotic foci.

An estrogen–progestogen combination and a progestogen alone can both be used successfully for temporary treatment of a generally severely symptomatic condition such as RVE. It causes a progressive, constant and substantial decrease in pain symtoms.[20] It causes minor variations in lipid profile.[20] The ethinyl estradiol plus cyproterone acetate combination is slightly less effective but well-tolerated, and could be suggested for women with acne or hypertrichosis and those who experience androgenic side effects with norethindrone acetate.[20]

The identification of safe and effective alternatives to prolong treatment constitutes an important part of research. The possibility of aiming the therapeutic action of drugs at specific organs, thus reducing general metabolic impact. Three different 'topical' options have been studied in women with RVE, namely, danazol-loaded vaginal ring, suppositories and capsules; intrauterine levonorgestrel (as a medicated IUD), and a contraceptive ring releasing an estrogen–progestin combination.[1]

Very recently Vercellini et al (2009a)[21] evaluated the efficacy and tolerability of a contraceptive vaginal ring and transdermal patch in the treatment of endometriosis-associated pain.

Inconvenience of the daily pill routine lead to use of a monthly vaginal ring and a weekly transdermal patch, that deliver the same types of hormone combinations used in OCs without requiring daily use providing greater convenience and the potential for superior tolerance and compliance.[21] Continuous administration maintains constant plasma drug levels and eliminates the peaks and troughs associated with oral administration. Loss of bioavailability, owing to first-pass hepatic metabolism and enzymatic degradation in the gastrointestinal tract observed in oral drug use, is prevented.[21] Finally, absorption is not influenced by episodes of vomiting or diarrhea. Vaginal discomfort was more common in ring users, whereas nausea, vomiting, headache, breast tenderness, and cutaneous reactions were more common in patch users. It causes major reduction in pain symptoms, probably similar to OCs.[21] It was very effective in dysmenorrhea. Deep dyspareunia decreased substantially.[1] Women who chose a contraceptive vaginal ring for the treatment of recurrent symptomatic endometriosis were significantly more satisfied than those who chose a contraceptive transdermal patch. The ring was more effective than patch in terms of pain reduction.[1] Both systems were associated with suboptimal results in terms of patient adherence. Neither delivery systems guaranteed sufficient bleeding control. Besides they are more expensive than the OCs.[21]

Danazol

Low-dose vaginal danazol is highly effective in the treatment of the painful symptoms associated with recurrent deeply infiltrating endometriosis, reducing the size of endometriotic lesions, and has no systemic side effects.[22]

Razzi et al (2007)[22] treated 21 patients with postoperative persistence of deeply infiltrating RVE with vaginal danazol capsules, 200 mg/day for

12 months. The subjective assessment of pain intensity by a visual analogue pain scale provided an adequate assessment of dysmenorrhea, dyspareunia, and pelvic pain, associated with an improved quality of life in these patients with deeply infiltrating endometriosis. The effect on organic symptoms may be due not only to the volumetric reduction of rectovaginal plaques but also most probably to reduced intralesional and perilesional inflammation and to reduced production of prostaglandins and cytokines, which stimulate pain fibers.

Vaginal danazol does not affect the menstrual cycle. It has few side effects and is not associated with an increase of protein S, protein C, and antithrombin in contrast with classical danazol treatment.[22]

It may be one of the new alternatives to repeat surgery in medical treatment of recurrent deeply infiltrating endometriosis.

It does not inhibit ovulation and may be highly teratogenic if conception occurs. Cost limits its feasibility for long-term use.

Danazol releasing vaginal rings have been tried. They have shown to decrease dysmenorrhea and size of lesions. However, ovarian endometriosis would be unresponsive to It.[19]

Levonorgestrel-Releasing Intrauterine Device (LNG-IUD)

Progestins have long been considered effective medical therapy for endometriosis.[19] In recent years, their role has been reaffirmed, because other modern therapies have the drawback of being expensive.[19] They have increased patient compliance during long-term treatments.[1] The introduction of a levonorgestrel-releasing IUD provides the option of hormonal treatment with a progestin, which is released locally at therapeutic concentrations and produces few systemic side effects.[19] It decreases pelvic pain symptoms caused by peritoneal and rectovaginal endometriosis and reduces the risk of recurrence of dysmenorrhea after conservative surgery, associated with local drug concentrations greater than plasma levels and limited adverse effects.[22] This T-shaped sylastic structure includes a reservoir positioned along the vertical arm that contains 52 mg of levonorgestrel. The release rate is 20 µg/day, and the device is left in place for at least 5 years.[19] Its mechanism of action is probably a receptor-mediated effect of levonorgestrel at the level of the endometriotic foci or secondary oligoamenorrhea and the consequent reduction in cyclic bleeding at ectopic endometrial sites.[19]

To evaluate the effectiveness of the LNG-IUD as a therapy for RVE, Fedele et al. (2001)[19] recruited 11 symptomatic women who had previously undergone conservative surgery without excision of deep lesions and assessed variations in pain symptoms and size of plaques.[1] Pain associated with endometriosis of the rectovaginal septum improved markedly.[19] There was a small but significant reduction in the volume of the lesions. It can have an important role in long-term management of pain associated with endometriosis in patients with no immediate desire to conceive.[19,22]

However recently, doubts have been expressed on the overall satisfaction and continuation rate in LNG-IUD users due to unscheduled bleeding, lower abdominal pain and progestogenic side effects.[1] More data and comparative trials are needed also to confirm the effect on dyspareunia and dyschezia and to verify whether the good results reported are maintained during the entire 5-year period of system efficacy.[1]

Gonadotrophin-Releasing Hormone Agonist (GnRH Agonist)

Fedele et al (2000)[23] evaluated the effect of treatment with leuprolide acetate, 3.75 mg IM/28 days for 6 months, in 15 women with symptomatic RVE, previously operated without excision of the deeply infiltrating lesion. They are successful but the side effects and cost usually limit the feasibility of prolonged use.

Some studies have used a preoperative course of GnRH agonist and found bleeding to be less and excision easier during surgery.

Aromatase Inhibitors

Aromatization (i.e. the conversion of C19 steroids to estrogens) is a very important step in estrogen formation. This reaction is catalyzed by the P450 aromatase mono-oxygenase enzyme complex, which is present in the smooth endoplasmic reticulum and functions as a demethylase. Increasing evidence suggests that endometrial aromatase expression is involved in the pathogenesis of endometriosis.[24]

Hefler et al (2005)[24] administered aromatase inhibitor anastrozole. They were found least encouraging.[1] Consequently Remorgida et al (2007b)[25] reported the results of a double drug regimen including the aromatase inhibitor letrozole (2.5 mg/day per os) and norethisterone acetate (2.5 mg/day per os). But based on the available information, the combination of an aromatase inhibitor in addition to a standard regimen does not seem an appropriate choice as a first-line treatment for RVE.[1]

In a review of literature on medical treatment for RVE, it was seen that with the exception of an aromatase inhibitor used alone, the antalgic effect of the considered medical therapies was high for the entire treatment period (from 6 to 12 months), with 60 to 90% of patients reporting considerable reduction or complete relief from pain symptoms.[1] Despite favorable results during treatment, pain recurrence was the rule at drug withdrawal and about half of the symptomatic patients evaluated at follow-up eventually underwent surgery.[1]

Surgical

Surgery is the first option in the treatment of endometriosis, and laparoscopy is the surgical technique that is most preferred **(Figs 14.7 to 14.14)**. Endometriosis is a disease of women in reproductive age; and in the majority of cases, one must

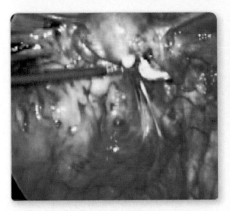

Figure 14.7: Rectovaginal endometriosis

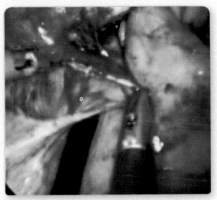

Figure 14.8: Identification of left ureter on laparoscopy

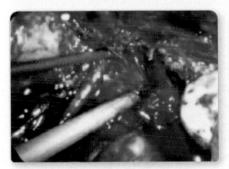

Figure 14.9: Left lateral window on laparoscopy

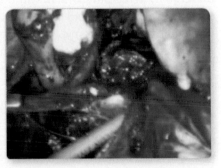

Figure 14.10: Left pararectal space created

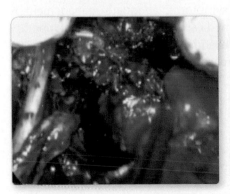

Figure 14.11: Rectovaginal nodule

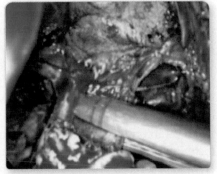

Figure 14.12: Rectosigmoid resection

maintain the fertility of the patient. The objectives of conservative surgical treatment of endometriosis are:

❖ Eradication of endometriotic lesions
❖ Preservation of ovarian function
❖ Relief of symptoms
❖ Limitation of recurrence.

The best results are achieved when surgical treatment is not conservative. Women with pain from

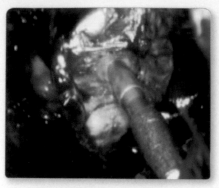

Figure 14.13: Anvil coupling

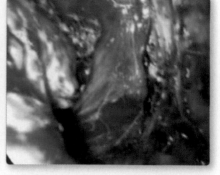

Figure 14.14: Anorectal anastomosis

endometriosis refractory to conservative, medical, or surgical therapy often undergo hysterectomy, with or without bilateral oophorectomy. Determinants such as age, gravidity, and parity must be considered when deciding whether to perform oophorectomy. Subtotal hysterectomy must be avoided because in a great number of patients with endometriosis, the cervix and uterosacral ligaments are involved in the disease. It is interesting to note the fact that hysterectomy is more successful for cyclic pelvic pain and when the pain is associated with uterine tenderness. Hormonal therapy is palliative, and the benefits are limited to the period of treatment.

Surgery, laparoscopic or laparotomic, must be performed depending on the extent and location of the disease. It is important to emphasize that, in advanced stages, laparoscopic or laparotomic surgery requires advanced surgical skills. A multidisciplinary approach often is needed.

As RVE causes such debilitating symptoms, adequate management is advocated. While hormone-based medical treatment allows temporary quiescence of active lesions[26,27] with subsequent short-term pain relief, several authors consider surgery, both laparoscopy and laparotomy, the optimal treatment for deep endometriosis, since it allows for the complete excision of the lesions and final diagnosis with successful long-term results.[28-33] Furthermore, it has been demonstrated that surgical treatment of deep endometriosis may improve the recovery of fertility.[34,35]

Several conservative surgical techniques have been proposed to deal with this technically demanding condition. Incomplete lesion resection generally does not achieve pain relief, whereas radical interventions carry the risk of major complications, and ureteral and rectal injuries with associated sequelae are not rare.

In the past few years, there has been considerable interest in elucidating the nature of deep and RVE in patients with pain, and in clarifying the appropriate surgical management to obtain prolonged amelioration of symptoms or cure. Medical suppressive therapy has been found to be either ineffective or temporary with high recurrence, whereas surgical excision is effective in relieving pain and dyspareunia symptoms and quality of life.

It has been stated that 'the definitive treatment of endometriosis is simple: surgical eradication' and that 'the success of surgical treatment is best assessed by determining how much disease, if any, remains after operative interventions'.[18]

Surgery is often considered the best treatment option in women with symptomatic endometriosis. However, extent and duration of the therapeutic benefit are still poorly defined. It became progressively evident that the overall 'amount' of disease is not correlated neither with frequency and severity of symptoms nor with long-term prognosis in terms of conceptions and pain recurrences.[18]

Excision of endometriotic lesions is a valid alternative in patients not responding to or not tolerating progestogens and estrogen-progestogen combinations. In particular, subjects suffering from severe deep dyspareunia and dyschezia should be considered good candidates, as removal of deep nodules is usually more effective than medical therapy in relieving organic-type pain. Finally, intolerable pain in women seeking a spontaneous conception constitutes a rational indication for conservative surgery.[18] Rectovaginal endometriosis invade deeply in the pelvic organs and the rectum, which require high surgical techniques and complete removal is extremely difficult. This goal of surgical completeness for endometriosis is even more difficult to attain when fertility is desired and the patient is symptomatic, because the preservation of the uterus may determine an incomplete removal of deep lesions.

For almost a century, the surgical treatment of endometriosis has been based mainly on a straightforward oncologic principle, i.e. radical removal of lesions. This is still a mainstay of therapy in cases of bowel and ureteral stenosis or adnexal masses with doubtful characteristics. However, even when this is not the case, many surgeons maintain that it is preferable undergoing a minimally invasive intervention than years of medications with the associated untoward effects. Moreover, conservative surgery is the only alternative in women seeking conception, as drugs used for endometriosis interfere with ovulation. Gynecologists advocating medical treatments argue that, in the majority of patients, control of pain is simple and effective with oral contraceptives or progestins. These hormones are safe, well-tolerated, inexpensive and can be used for years, thus limiting the costs and morbidity of multiple surgical procedures. According to this view, laparoscopy should be limited to non-responders as well as symptomatic women wishing to achieve a pregnancy spontaneously. Because none of the above approaches is curative and both have advantages and disadvantages, the two positions coexist and the debate continues. Very few RCT on surgery for endometriosis have been published. When considering the expected effect of surgery for endometriosis-associated pain, clinicians and patients should be aware that the outcome is operator-dependent.[18]

Surgical Treatment of RVE

Bowel preparation was done in all patients with suspected rectovaginal lesions. Two days before surgery, the patients followed a clear liquid diet and the morning before the surgery patients had exelyte liquid 45 ml in 300 ml of lime juice. On both days of liquid diet, patients were given Syp Duphalac 2 tsp at bedtime. This ensured that the bowel was well-prepared for the surgery.

All patients who had operative laparoscopy were operated on according to the following technique. After the induction of pneumoperitoneum (Achieved by insertion of veress needle at Palmer's point) and introduction of the laparoscopic fiber optic and two or three ancillary ports, the pelvis was inspected and cleared of adhesions. Adhesiolysis and dissection were performed with laparoscopic scissors, and hemostasis was ensured by performing adhesiolysis in the correct plane. Bipolar coagulation was used to the bare minimum. After adhesiolysis, the deep endometriotic implants were dissected and isolated, then removed. Dissection was carried out until the loose areolar tissue of the retroperitoneal space was reached.

In patients in whom the rectal wall was involved, a careful dissection was done until the normal muscularis layers of the rectum were reached. When necessary, ureterolysis and dissection of the lateral rectal space were carried out. Ureters were always identified before proceeding to dissection of deep implants infiltrating uterosacral ligaments. Endometriosis infiltrating the whole thickness of the vaginal wall through the mucosa required partial colpectomy combined with rectovaginal septum dissection. Associated endometriotic lesions (i.e. ovarian cysts, superficial peritoneal implants, adnexal adhesions) were treated during the same operative procedures, following the technique previously described.

'Rectal endometriosis' was defined as being deep posterior endometriosis involving muscular, submucosal or mucosal layers of the rectum, up to 13 cm from the anus, indicated by MRI and endorectal ultrasound examination, and later intraoperatively confirmed.

Surgical treatment of rectal endometriosis may be a difficult choice as patients are young, professionally active and plan to conceive.[5] Several types of surgery are performed for severe endometriosis involving the bowel. Whereas debulking, leaving some endometriosis on the bowel in order to avoid opening the bowel, seems to have lost popularity, it remains unclear whether and when a discoid or segmental bowel resection should be performed. Randomized trials comparing outcome are not and will not be available shortly for the obvious reasons that series are too small and that surgeons who are equally skilled in both procedures are rare. The argument in favor of segmental bowel resection is completeness of endometriosis removal, especially if the area affected is larger than 2 cm.[36-38]

Role of Robotics

Using a computer generated robotic system has multiple advantages. It provides a 3 dimensional view, excellent visualization of the surgical field and tremor free movements. The surgical protocol varies according to the lesion, its location, extent and symptomatology, but inherently it is standardized.

❖ Bowel preparation (preoperative)
❖ Identification of both ureters at pelvic brim and dissection with lateralization from normal, through diseased to normal anatomy
❖ Vaginal entry into bilateral pararectal fossae with exteriorization of vaginal wall endometriosis for partial colpectomy later on
❖ Mobilization of rectosigmoid upto rectovaginal fascia
❖ Dissection and cephalation of affected segment from uterine cervix and posterior uterine wall through large amount of surrounding fibrosis
❖ Nerve identification and preservation of plexus
❖ Division of mesocolon in anticipation of division of rectal wall
❖ Use of endo GIA to divide rectum at the disease free margin
❖ Postcolpotomy to deliver the proximal rectum and completion of proximal division with purse string (interlocking) suture to introduce part of end to end anastomosis stapler followed by redeposition of proximal rectum
❖ Introduction of end to end anastomosis stapler per rectally
❖ Anastomosis of rectal stump to sigmoid colon using the circular stapler
❖ Air insufflations under pressure to assure there is no leak.

The recent advent of computer enhanced robotic technology more sophisticated instruments and better energy sources may provide the bridge necessary for surgeons to incorporate laparoscopic surgery into their practices, cost being only deterrent.

If you can see more and see better you can do more and do better.

Major complications are observed in 3 to 10% of the patients, including hemoperitoneum, rectovaginal fistula, anastomotic leakage/fistula, ureteral fistula/uroperitoneum, bowel perforation, pelvic abscess, need for temporary loop ileostomy, postoperative bowel or ureteral anastomotic stenosis, neurogenic bladder dysfunction, constipation and peripheral sensory disturbance. Excision of the posterior vaginal fornix was associated with substantial pain reduction (particularly deep dyspareunia), but concomitant resection of vaginal and rectal walls increased the likelihood of fistula formation due to juxtaposition of sutures of bacteria-containing hollow viscera.[18]

For bowel resections performed for deep endometriosis, low leakage rates and organ dysfunction rates are reported in various studies, but the numbers remain small.

Postoperative leakage: The overall incidence of anastomostic leak rate after colorectal resection was reported to have a wide variation in the different studies. These large differences may be explained at least partially by surgeon experience, as concluded by Chambers et al. Indeed, experienced surgeons had a rate between 3.4% and 6%.[36] The lower the anastomosis, the higher the probability of postoperative leakage. It has been consistently reported that leakage was more common after anterior resections, especially for low resections less than 7 cm from the anal verge.[36,37] For sigmoid resections, rates varied between 0 to 2.9%; while for anterior resections, these values varied between 0 to 12.7%.[36,38]

Stapled Vs hand sewn anastomosis: Several trials addressed the differences between stapled anastomosis and hand-sewn anastomosis. Some confusion persists as endoscopic surgery preferentially uses stapled anastomosis. After open surgery, no difference in leak rates was found, as concluded in a Cochrane review meta-analysis of 9 randomized trials[39] that compared the results of 622 stapled versus 611 hand-sewn anastomoses. Also,Kockerling et al reported anastomotic leak rates of 4.7% with stapled anastomoses versus 3.2% in the hand-sewn group, whereas Mileski et al found no difference, with rates of 4.4% and 3.5%, respectively.[37,40] After stapled anastomosis, we found leak rates between 1.6% and 4.25% versus 0 to 6% for those reports with predominantly hand-sewn anastomosis in various studies.

Low Vs high resection: Although laparoscopic colorectal resection is considered feasible and safe,[38] there is agreement that this type of procedure should be performed by only experienced colorectal surgeons. Moreover, the lower the anterior resection, the greater the technical difficulties in resections. For benign conditions, leak rates after sigmoid resections should be around 1%. Clinical diagnosis may be difficult, supporting those who advocate a liberal use of imaging techniques when in doubt or a repeat laparoscopy when a leak is strongly suspected. The incidence of functional bowel problems, as well as urinary and sexual problems, up to 30% and even 40% is high, especially after low rectum resections.

Functional outcome: The functional results after intestinal resection for benign conditions rarely have been reported. Most studies describe outcomes after resection for malignant disease, which probably is radical, with more autonomic nerve injury and frequently with neoadjuvant radiotherapy. Autonomic nerve damage is the most likely cause of sexual and urinary dysfunction.

Bladder and sexual dysfunction are well-known sequelae of rectal surgery as they usually occur as a result of damage of the autonomic nerves. With the advent of new techniques that aim at preservation of nerve structures, these complications will decrease.

Important Facts Regarding Surgical Management

Anastomostic leakage is a feared complication of colorectal surgery and if unrecognized may be associated with a mortality as high as 39%.

Leak incidence and bowel dysfunction are clearly more common after lower resections. It was suggested to be secondary to a low blood supply in the lower part of the rectum, affecting anastomostic healing.

Functional bowel problems occur less often after sigmoid than after rectum resection. These problems were reported to be related to the length of residual rectum, which is considered of crucial importance for normal function. The surgical technique is also vital however the difference with different techniques has not been assessed in a randomized study.

Urogenital dysfunction after bowel resection is generally explained by anatomy, especially the sympathetic and parasympathetic nerve supply. Because the pelvic autonomic nerve plexus is localized in the anterolateral area of the rectum, the probability of damage is higher in low resections.

Functional problems reported after endometriosis surgery involved mainly urinary retention, a consequence of parasympathetic damage that is related more often to the lateral extent of the endometriosis.

Finally, although laparoscopic colorectal resection is considered feasible and safe, there is agreement that this type of procedure should be performed by only experienced colorectal surgeons. Clearly there is marked improvement in the quality of life in patients with rectovaginal endometriosis after bowel resection.

Complications

❖ Persistence of pain.
❖ Recurrence of pain
❖ Quality of life hampered.
❖ Ureteral stenosis
❖ Surgery related complications.

Malignant changes are rare. Most tumors are of epithelial origin, are endometrioid carcinoma and clear cell carcinoma. Rare cases of stromal neoplasms including adenocarcinoma have been reported.[41]

Ureteral endometriosis is infrequent, accounting for less than 0.3% of all endometriotic lesions. Ureteral lesions are relatively rare but serious because they may cause silent loss of renal function.[42]

➲ FERTILITY AND RVE

Most endometriosis patients have problems of infertility. Inspite of the advances in the field of assisted reproduction fertility outcome remains unsatisfactory. Laparoscopic treatment also has a questionable efficiency with regard to achieving better fertility results, with controversies mainly surrounding ovarian residual reserve.

Outcomes in assisted reproduction techniques (ART) in endometriosis remain unsatisfactory, revealing impaired pregnancy and implantation rates in comparison with infertility due to tubal or male factors. Pregnancy rates after laparoscopic procedure for RVE treatment varies. There is no homogeneity among the studies and comparison of pregnancy rates between those after surgery and those who underwent ART remain to be analyzed.

⊃ REFERENCES

1. Vercillini P, Crosignani PG, Somigliana E, Berlanda N, Barbara G, Fedele L. Medical treatment for rectovaginal endometriosis: what is the evidence? Hum Reprod 2009;24(10):2504-14.
2. Guerriero S, Ajossa S, Gerada M, Virgilio B, Angioni S, Melis GB. Diagnostic value of transvaginal 'tenderness-guided' ultrasonography for the prediction of location of deep endometriosis. Hum. Reprod. 2008;23(11):2452–7.
3. Carmona F, Martinez-Zamora A, Gonzalez X, Gines A, Bunesch L, Balasch J. Does the learning curve of conservative laparoscopic surgery in women with rectovaginalendometriosis impair the recurrence rate? Fertil and Steril. 2009;92(3):868-75.
4. Menada MV, Remorgida V, Abbamonte LH, Nicoletti A, Ragni N, Ferrero S. Does transvaginal ultrasonography combined with water-contrast in the rectum aid in the diagnosis of rectovaginal endometriosis infiltrating the bowel? Hum Reprod. 2008;23(5):1069-75.
5. Roman H, Loisel C, Resch B, Tuech J.J, Hochain P, Leroi AM, et al. Delayed functional outcomes associated with surgical management of deep rectovaginal endometriosis with rectal involvement: giving patients an informed choice. Hum Reprod. 2010;25(4): 890–9.
6. Dessole S, Farina M, Rubattu G, Cosmi E, Ambrosin G, Nardelli GB. Sonovaginography is a new technique for assessing rectovaginal endometriosis. Fertil and Steril 2003;79(4):1023-7.
7. Forda J, Englisha J, Milesb WA, Giannopoulosa T. Pain, quality of life and complications following the radical resection of rectovaginal endometriosis. BJOG: an Int J Obstet and Gynaec. 2004;111:353-6.
8. Parazzini F, Cipriani S, Moroni S, Crosignani PG. Relationship between stage, site and morphological characteristics of pelvic endometriosis and pain. Hum Reprod 2001;16(12):2668-71.
9. Redwine DB. Laparoscopicen bloc resection for treatment of the obliterated cul-de-sac in endometriosis. J Reprod Med. 1992;37:695-8.
10. Pascual MA, Guerriero S, Hereter L, Barri-Soldevila P, Ajossa S, et al. Diagnosis of endometriosis of the rectovaginal septum using introital three-dimensional ultrasonography. Fertil and Steril. 2010;94(7):2761-5.
11. Bazot M, Lafont C, Rouzier R, Roseau G, Thomassin-Naggara I, Darai E. Diagnostic accuracy of physical examination, transvaginal sonography, rectal endoscopic sonography, and magnetic resonance imaging to diagnose deep infiltrating endometriosis. Fertil and Steril. 2009;92(6):1825-33.
12. Menada MV, Remorgida V, Abbamonte LH, Fulcheri E, Ragni N, Ferrero S. Transvaginal ultrasonography combined with water-contrast in the rectum in the diagnosis of rectovaginal endometriosis infiltrating the bowel. Fertil and Steril 2008;89(3):699-700.
13. Bazot M, Bornier C, Dubernard G, Roseau G, Cortez A, Dara E. Accuracy of magnetic resonance imaging and rectal endoscopic sonography for the prediction of location of deep pelvic endometriosis. Hum Reprod. 2007;22(5):1457–63.
14. Kinkel K, Chapron C, Balleyguier C, Fritel X, Dubuisson JB, Moreau JF. Magnetic resonance imaging characteristics of deep endometriosis. Hum Reprod. 1999; 14(4):1080–6.
15. Chapron C, Vieira M, Chopin N, Balleyguier C, Barakat H, Dumontier I, et al. Accuracy of rectal endoscopic ultrasonography and magnetic resonance imaging in the diagnosis of rectal involvement for patients presenting with deeply infiltrating endometriosis. Ultrasound Obstet Gynecol 2004;24:175–9.

16. Takeuchi H, Kuwatsuru R, Kitade M, Sakurai A, Kikuchi I, et al. A novel technique using magnetic resonance imaging jelly for evaluation of rectovaginal endometriosis. Fertil and Steril. 2005;83(2):442-7.
17. Koninckx PR, Martin D. Treatment of deeply infiltrating endometriosis. Curr Opin Obstet Gynecol. 1994;6:231-41.
18. Vercellini P, Crosignani PG, Abbiati A, Somigliana E, Vigano P, Fedele L. The effect of surgery for symptomatic endometriosis: the other side of the story. Hum Reprod 2009;15(2):177–88.
19. Fedele L, Bianchi S, Zanconato G, Portuese A, Raffaelli R. Use of a levonorgestrel-releasing intrauterine device in the treatment of rectovaginal endometriosis. Fertil and Steril. 2001;75(3):485-8.
20. Vercellini P, Pietropaolo G, Giorgi OD, Pasin R, Chiodini A, Crosignani PG. Treatment of symptomatic rectovaginal endometriosis with an estrogen–progestogen combination versus low-dose norethindrone acetate. Fertil and Steril 2005; 84(5):1375-87.
21. Vercillini P, Barbara G, Somigliana E, Bianchi S, Abbiati A, Fedele L. Comparison of contraceptivering and patch for the treatment of symptomatic endometriosis. Fertil and Steril. 2010;93(7):2150-61.
22. Razzi S, Luisi S, Calonaci F, Altomare A, Bocchi C, Petraglia F. Efficacy of vaginaldanazol treatment in women with recurrent deeply infiltrating endometriosis. Fertil and Steril. 2007;88(4):789-94.
23. Fedele L, Bianchi S, Zanconato G, Tozzi L, Raffaelli R. Gonadotropin-releasing hormone agonist treatment for endometriosis of the rectovaginal septum. Am J Obstet Gynecol. 2000;183:1462-7.
24. Hefler LA, Grimm C, Trotsenburg MV, Nagele F. Role of the vaginally administered aromatase inhibitor anastrozole in women with rectovaginal endometriosis: a pilot study. Fertil and Steril. 2005;84(4):1033-6.
25. Remorgida V, Abbamonte HL, Ragni N, Fulcheri E, Ferrero S. Letrozole and norethisterone acetate in rectovaginal endometriosis. Fertil and Steril 2007; 88(3):724-6.
26. Brosens IA, Verleyen A, Cornillie F. The morphologic effect of short-term medical therapy of endometriosis. Am J Obstet Gynecol.1987;157:1215-21.
27. Nisolle-Pochet M, Casanas-Roux F, Donnez J. Histologic study of ovarian endometriosis after hormonal therapy. Fertil Steril. 1988;49:423-6.
28. Nezhat C, Nezhat F, Pennington E. Laparoscopic treatment of infiltrative rectosigmoid colon and rectovaginal septum endometriosis by the technique of videolaparoscopy and the CO_2 laser. Br J Obstet Gynaecol. 1992;99:664-7.
29. Reich H, McGlynn F, Salvat J. Laparoscopic treatment of cul-de-sac obliteration secondary to retrocervical deep fibrotic endometriosis. J Reprod Med. 1991;36: 516-22.
30. Redwine DB. Conservative laparoscopic excision of endometriosis by sharp dissection: life-table analysis of reoperation and persistent or recurrent disease. Fertil Steril. 1991;56:628-34.
31. Chapron C, Dubuisson DB, Fritel X, et al. Operative management of deep endometriosis infiltrating the uterosacral ligaments. J Am Assoc Gynecol Laparosc. 1999;6:31-7.
32. Crosignani PG, Vercellini P. Conservative surgery for severe endometriosis: should laparotomy be abandoned definitively? Hum Reprod.1995;10:2412-8.
33. Crosignani PG, Vercellini P, Biffignandi F, et al. Laparoscopy versus laparotomy in conservative surgical treatment for severe endometriosis. Fertil Steril. 1996;66: 706-11.

34. Chapron C, Fritel X, Dubuisson DB. Fertility after laparoscopic management of deep endometriosis infiltrating uterosacral ligaments. Hum Reprod. 1999;14:329-32.
35. Redwine DB, Wright JT. Laparoscopic treatment of complete obliteration of the cul-de-sac associated with endometriosis: long-term follow-up of en bloc resection. Fertil Steril. 2001;76:358-65.
36. Nezhat C, Nezhat F, Pennington E. Laparoscopic treatment of infiltrative recto-sigmoid colon and rectovaginal septum endometriosis by the technique of video laparoscopy and the CO_2 laser. BJOG. 1992;99:664–7.
37. Jerby BL, Kessler H, Falcone T, et al. Laparoscopic management of colorectal endometriosis. Surg Endosc. 1999;13:1125–8.
38. Possover M, Diebolder H, Plaul K, et al. Laparoscopically assisted vaginal resection of rectovaginal endometriosis. Obstet Gynecol. 2000;96:304 –7.
39. Lustosa SAS, Matos D, Atallah AN, et al. Stapled versus hand-sewn methods for colorectal anastomosis surgery. Cochrane Database Syst Rev. 2001;3:CD003144.
40. Mileski WJ, Joehi RJ, Rege RV, et al. Treatment of anastomostic leakage following low anterior colon resection. Arch Surg. 1988;123:968–71.
41. Raffaelli R, Piazzola E, Zanconato G, Fedele L. A rare case of extrauterine adeno-sarcoma arising in endometriosis of the rectovaginal septum. Fertil and Steril 2004;81(4):1142-4.
42. Donnez J, Nisolle M, Squifflet J. Ureteral endometriosis: a complication of rectovaginal endometriotic (adenomyotic) nodules. Fertil and Steril 2002; 77(1): 32-7.

Coping Up with Endometriosis

◀ Sujata Kar

➲ INTRODUCTION

Defined as the presence of endometrial-like glands and stroma in any extra uterine site, endometriosis occurs in 6 to 22% of women of reproductive age women. It is a huge global burden, as approximately 176 million women worldwide are affected by it regardless of their ethnic or social status and many more, who go undiagnosed. Women suffer with a range of signs and symptoms and for physicians the endometriosis disease is a challenge.

➲ ENDOMETRIOSIS: AN ENIGMA

Each month a woman's ovaries produce hormones that stimulate the cells of the uterine lining (endometrium) to multiply and prepare for a fertilized egg. If these cells (called endometrial cells) grow outside the uterus, endometriosis results. Unlike cells normally found in the uterus that are shed during menstruation, the ones outside the uterus stay in place. They sometimes bleed a little bit, but they heal and are stimulated again during the next cycle. This ongoing process leads to symptoms of endometriosis (pain) and can cause scars (adhesions) on the tubes, ovaries, and surrounding structures in the pelvis. It has been suggested that virtually all women are potentially vulnerable to the development of the lesions of endometriosis, but appropriate immunocompetency in most eradicates such lesions in a timely fashion, preventing clinical sequelae. The most common sites for endometrial implantation within the pelvis are the ovaries, broad and round ligaments, fallopian tubes, cervix, vagina and pouch of Douglas **(Table 15.1)**. The gastrointestinal tract may be involved in about 12% of cases and the urinary tract is affected in about 1%.
In-fact "endometriosis" can affect just about any tissue or organ.

Table 15.1: Risk factor for developing endometriosis

•	Reproductive age
•	Early menarche
•	Prolonged and frequent cycles
•	Nullipara
•	Cryptomenorrhea
•	Family history

The Impact of Endometriosis

The 'impact' that a disease like endometriosis has on women health, work and psychology has rarely been appreciated.

Doctors, family, employers need to understand this painful condition and have a sympathetic attitude towards it.

In an unique, unprecedented move, endometriosis was addressed at a legislative level in the united states, during the "women in Government's" 2nd Annual Healthcare Summit, in Washington DC in Nov 2011.

The World Endometrisis Research Foundation's (WERF) chief executive Lone Hommelsho emphasized few important points:

1. Endometriosis affects women's general, physical, social and mental well-being during their prime and most productive decades.
2. It is not a "life style disease". It does not discriminate between age, ethnic or social circumstances.
3. Affects an estimated 176 million women and girls world wide.
4. She presented preliminary data from WERF's endocost study which suggests that reduced productivity at work by women with painful endometriosis may account for twice that of direct heath care costs—all because of the pain associated with the disease preventing these women to perform optimally.
5. First global studies investigating impact and cost of endometriosis, across ten countries on five continents report a 38% greater loss of work productivity.
6. Most women are diagnosed late, more than 7 years on an average, inspite of presenting with symptoms suggestive of endometriosis.
7. Presented suggestions as to what can be done at "legislative level"
   - Education of young women and primary care providers, about menstrual pain and the disease
   - Specialist care and appropriate reimbursement should be available
   - Funding and greater emphasis on research into disease mechanisms.

➲ DIAGNOSIS

Symptoms often do not correleate well with the stage of endometriosis. The criterion standard for the diagnosis of endometriosis is still considered by most to be direct visualization by laparoscopy or histologic findings or both.

The cause of endometriosis is unknown, only there are a number of theories.

Endometriosis is a condition in which the tissue that behaves like the cells lining the uterus (endometrium) grows in other areas of the body, causing pain, irregular bleeding, and possible infertility .The tissue growth (implant) typically occurs in the pelvic area, outside of the uterus, on the ovaries, bowel, rectum, bladder, and the delicate lining of the pelvis. However, the implants can occur in other areas of the body, too. Typically, "Pain" is the main symptom for women with endometriosis. This can include:

❖ Painful periods
❖ Pain in the lower abdomen or pelvic cramps that can be felt for a week or two before menstruation
❖ Pain in the lower abdomen felt during menstruation (the pain and cramps may be steady and dull or severe)
❖ Pain during or following sexual intercourse
❖ Pain with bowel movements
❖ Pelvic or low back pain that may occur at any time during the menstrual cycle.

Thus, most common symptoms: persistent pelvic pain, dyspareunia, dyschezia, dysmenorrhea, bloating, acne, diarrhea, constipation, infertility, pelvic /ovarian masses. Often, there are no symptoms. In fact, some women with severe cases of endometriosis have no pain at all, whereas some women with mild endometriosis have severe pain **(Table 15.2)**.

Table 15.2: Treatment options

Medical	Surgical
Analgesics, OCPs, progestins, GnRH analogues, Mirena	Type of surgery, extent, radical, conservative, laparoscopic, laparotomy

Therefore, peculiarity of this disease is *"severity of symptoms often do not match extent of the disease"*.

How to Cope with Endometriosis?

Coping with endometriosis means "living with endometriosis".

It is a chronic ailment and therefore a life-long battle for most women. Endometriosis is a significant health problem for women of reproductive age and claims lot of work hours.

Women need to understand the disease to be able to deal with it.

Many women with endometriosis will have to accept that they have to learn to live with and manage chronic pain, deal with infertility, and other such issues, because everybody will not be fortunate enough to find a cure or a remission.

There is no single prescription or blue print for coping. People use a number of different ways to cope, different methods work for different individuals, and some may wish to consult different health care providers for supportive treatment, for example—psysiotherapists/counselors/psychologists/nutritionists, etc.

Some Coping Tips

1. **Consultation**
   Involves two steps
   a. First is to find the correct physician who understands the disease and is compassionate to the women's symptoms.

- It can be difficult to find a doctor who has all the following qualifications:
  * Thorough knowledge of endometriosis
  * Surgical skills
  * Current understanding of various treatments
  * Openness to complementary approaches
  * Compassion for the patient's symptoms
  * Ready to refer to another expert if the need be
  * These traits might be beyond a family doctor or even a typical gynecologist
  * Curently there is no gynecological sub-specialty called "Endometriosis expert" although there probably should be
  * Finding an expert physician early can help prevent delayed diagnosis, misdiagnosis, inadequate treatment, stress and wasted effort.

b. Second is to be able to communicate effectively with your doctor. To be able to express your symptoms accurately only then can a doctor appreciate the extent of the suffering.
  - It is a good plan to think and write down the major complaints before the doctor's appointment. Go over the questions and complaints in your mind before meeting the doctor. This way one can remain focused on the objective. Do not be vogue, but specific about your complains.

2. **Coping with the treatment**
Obviously, treatment has to be decided by the physician. Which may be medical or surgical. Generally neither of which are free of side effects, and have a prolonged recovery.
  - Some tips for dealing with side effects associated with drug treatments
  - With the drug treatments for endometriosis, the women's body goes into a state of "artificial menopause" that can have few unpleasant side effects. Hot flushes and night sweats can be very disturbing and interfere with work and sleep. Some tips:
    * Eat a healthy diet consisting of fresh vegetables whole grains, fresh fruit and the good fat found in fish, olive oil and nuts
    * Avoid refined sugar, flour and processed foods
    * Avoid alcoholic drugs, hot drinks can also trigger a hot flash (caffeine)
    * Avoid spicy food
    * Drink plenty of water
    * Dress lightly, use natural fibric like cotton, silk, linen
    * Do some from of physical exercise regularly. Research shows that regular exercise reduces the severity of hot flushes
    * Avoid smoking
    * Try relaxation techniques, meditation ,yoga. Reduction in stress levels can reduce severity of symptoms.

    * Supplements that may help are vitamin E, evening primrose oil, viatmin B complex, calcium and magnesium.
    * Add back therapy prescribed can also help alleviate many symptoms associated with therapy.

Golden rule is to find the right surgeon and laparoscopy for all cases.

3. **Nutrition and diet**: A nutritious and balanced diet is necessary for all aspects of "healthy living". However an endometriosis diet may be considered. Omit caffeine, alcohol, red meat, fatty fried food and animal fat. Add foods rich in omega 3 fatty acids, green leafy vegetables, fruit, whole grain. Opt for organic food. Avoid constipation.

4. **Physical activity**: Exercise releases endorphins which are natural pain killers. Reduces stress. Get adequate sleep.

5. **Lifestyle issues:** Simplify life, learn relaxation techniques, positive attitude to life and its problems, etc. may sound repetitive, but their importance cannot be undermined.

6. **Support groups**: A lot of emotional and physical stress can be handled by talking to women with similar problems. One can create ones own support group amongst friends and relatives with this disease or join a internet group. National support organizations in many countries, online support and chat groups exist. You can register for online endometriosis news, links to resources for endometriosis.

7. **Self-help books**.

Global forums
• www.endometriosis.org
• Endometriosis community on facebook.
• World endometriosis society
• World endometriosis research foundation

Common myths about endometriosis
• Menstrual pain is normal
• Teenagers and very young women are unlikely to have endometriosis
• Pregnancy cures endometriosis
• Surgery cures endometriosis
• Hormonal treatment cures endometriosis
• It is not possible to conceive with endometriosis
• Lot of endometriosis means lot of pain

➲ CONCLUSION

Awareness of endometriosis as a disease with substantial morbidity is of vital importance. Knowledge and skill for treating laparoscopy is increasingly becoming an area of subspecialization.

Endometriosis is a long-term condition. Many women have symptoms that occur off and on until menopause. Keep in mind that there are treatment options. A woman can work with her doctor to decide which treatment is right for her.

It also may help to talk with other women who are coping with endometriosis. Ask your doctor or nurse to suggest a support group in your area.

➲ SUGGESTED READING

1. Articles "Endometriosis.org" global forum on news and information about endometriosis.
2. Nnoaham KE, et al. Impact of endometriosis on quality of life and work productivity: a multicenter study across ten countries. Fertil.steril, 2011; 96(2):366.73.
3. Prost AM, lauter MR. Endometriosis in adolescents, incidence, diagnosis and treatment. T Reprod Med. 1999;44(9):751–8.
4. The endometriosis natural treatment program: A complete help plan for improving health and well being. Valerie Ann wormwood, Julia stonehouse.
5. The Endometriosis source book by Mary lou Ballweg.

Recent Advances of Treatment in Endometriosis

◀ Kamini A Rao, Mekala D

➲ INTRODUCTION

Endometriosis is defined as the presence of endometrial-like tissue outside the uterus, which induces a chronic, inflammatory reaction. The condition is predominantly found in women of reproductive age, from all ethnic and social groups.

Treatment must be individualized, taking the clinical problem in its entirety into account, including the impact of the disease and the effect of its treatment on quality of life. Pain symptoms may persist despite seemingly adequate medical and/or surgical treatment of the disease. In such circumstances, a multidisciplinary approach involving a pain clinic and counseling should be considered early in the treatment plan.

The following symptoms can be caused by endometriosis based on clinical and patient experience:

❖ Severe dysmenorrhea
❖ Deep dyspareunia
❖ Chronic pelvic pain
❖ Ovulation pain
❖ Cyclical or perimenstrual symptoms (e.g. bowel or bladder associated) with or without abnormal bleeding
❖ Infertility
❖ Chronic fatigue.

➲ TREATMENT OF ENDOMETRIOSIS ASSOCIATED PAIN

Nonsteroidal Anti-inflammatory Drugs

There is inconclusive evidence to show whether NSAIDs (specifically naproxen) are effective in managing pain caused by endometriosis.

Hormonal Treatment

A. *Progestagens*: Considered as a first choice for the treatment of endo-metriosis. There is no evidence that any single agent or any particular dose is preferable to another. In most studies, the effect of treatment has been evaluated after 3 to 6 months of therapy.

Other progestagens, such as desogestrel, are now being looked at as alternative treatments. The levonorgestrel intrauterine system (LNG-IUS) reduces endometriosis associated pain.

B. *COCs*: Cyclic regimen to women with endometriosis was found as effective as GnRH agonist treatment for relief of dyspareunia and nonmenstrual pain as assessed by a pain scoring system continuous low-dose OCs were more effective than cyclic OCs in controlling endometriosis symptoms in patients after surgical treatment for endometriosis medroxyprogesterone acetate (MPA), dydrogesterone, or norethindrone acetate, pain has been reduced by 70% to 100%.

C. *GnRH agonists*: Treatment for 3 months with a GnRH agonist may be as effective as 6 months in terms of pain relief.

D. *Danazole*: Proved to be effective in pain management; side effects prevent it from becoming a favorable option.

E. *Antiprogesterones*
  i. Gestrinone
  ii. MIfepristone these agents induce chronic anovulation and thereby reduce pain.

● NEWER TREATMENT MODALITIES

1. *The COC patch*: The patch is a type of hormone therapy that looks like a square adhesive bandage. It contains hormone medicine similar to birth control pills and is worn on the skin. Each hormone patch lasts one week. After 3 weeks of usage there would be a patch free week.

2. *The vaginal ring*: The vaginal ring is a small, thin, flexible rubber ring that fits inside the vagina. Once in place it releases a combination of estrogen and progestin (hormones). Similar to OCP's and the patch, the vaginal ring may be used to treat symptoms of endometriosis by controlling your menstrual cycle. Like the patch, this is also used cyclically.

3. *GnRH antagonist*: GnRH antagonists have been used for the treatment of pelvic endometriosis. However, they have not been as widely accepted as GnRH agonists.

4. *Aromatase inhibitors*: Aromatase enzyme is a target for selective inhibition of estrogen synthesis. The inhibition of local estrogen production in endometriotic implants is an attractive option for the management of endometriosis. The main side effects are hot flashes and gastrointestinal side effects.

5. *SPRMs*: SPRMs suppress estrogen-dependent endometrial growth and induce reversible amenorrhea. Progesterone treatment commonly causes breakthrough bleeding by inducing fragility of the endometrial blood vessels. SPRMs have the spiral arterioles as the target and causing stabilization of the endometrial blood vessels.

6. *SERMs*: Ormeloxifene has been tried. Larger studies are required to prove anything.
7. *Therapies under trail*
   a. *Antiangiogenesis therapy*: Antiangiogenesis therapy has been investigated in rodents, and Nap et al. (2005) demonstrated that angiostatic agents prevent the development of endometriosis-like lesions in the chicken chorioallantoic membrane. The future challenge is to successfully utilize it in women suffering from pelvic endometriosis.
   b. *Immunomodulators*: Four compounds with immune-enhancing properties have been investigated cytokines, interleukin-12 and interferon a-2b, and two synthetic immunomodulators, the guanosine analog loxoribine and the acetyl-choline nicotinic receptor agonist levamisole. Badawy et al demonstrated that interferon a-2b inhibits endometrioma cell growth in culture. D_Hooghe et al demonstrated that recombinant tumor necrosis factor–binding protein 1 inhibited the development of experimentally induced endometriosis in the baboon model. Keenan et al demonstrated the regression of experimentally induced endometriosis in rats using intraperitoneal loxoribine.
   c. *Chinese berbal medicine*: Although clinical studies on herbs in the literature show promising effects, conclusive clinical evidence of the efficacy of medicinal herbs in the treatment of endometriosis-associated pain is lacking.
   d. *VEGF-targeted CRADs*: In addition, the virus showed a similarly low tropism to the liver and eutopic endometrium *in vitro* and in a mouse model. In a clinical setting, VEGF-targeted CRADs could be administered into the abdominal cavity after laparoscopic resection of deep infiltrating endometriosis. Conditionally replicative adenoviruses (CRADs) designed Ad5VEGFE1 is a promising candidate for treating endometriosis and holds potential for clinical testing.

⟳ SURGICAL TREATMENT

Indications for surgical treatment:
* Pain
* Infertility
* Impaired bladder or ureteric function
* Impaired GI function.

Role of Surgery in Adolescents

Endometriosis should be considered in adolescents presenting with bilateral complex ovarian masses regardless of their size.

Laparoscopy should be considered if adolescents with chronic pelvic pain who do not respond to medical treatment (NSAIDs, OCPs) since endometriosis is very common under these circumstances. Minimal to mild endometriosis according to the rASRM classification are the most common stages of the disease in adolescents. Gynecologic surgeons should pay special attention to red, clear or white lesions which were reported to be more prevalent in adolescents as opposed to adults who have endometriosis. Menstrual outflow obstructions such as Müllerian anomalies may cause early development of endometriosis in adolescents. Regression of the disease has been observed once surgical correction of the anomaly has been accomplished. Physicians treating adolescents with endometriosis should adopt a multidimensional approach: surgery, hormonal manipulation, pain medication, mental health support, complementary and alternative therapies, and education in self-management strategies are useful components.

⊃ SURGERY IN REPRODUCTIVE AGE GROUP

Surgical Treatment for Endometriosis Associated Pain

Ideal practice is to diagnose and remove endometriosis surgically. Depending upon the severity of disease found, ideal practice is to diagnose and remove endometriosis surgically, provided that adequate preoperative consent has been obtained.

Peritoneal Lesions

Diagnostic laparoscopy without complete removal of endometriosis has been found to alleviate pain in 50% of patients.

Surgical options for the treatment of endometriosis include the use of unipolar or bipolar cautery, laser ablation using KTP, CO_2, or neodymium: yittrium, aluminum, garnet (Nd:YAG) lasers, and excision techniques, but no randomized trials have evaluated their comparative efficacies. Each has advantages .and disadvantages with respect to lesion removal, tissue trauma and bleeding.

Ablation of endometriotic lesions reduces endometriosis-associated pain compared with diagnostic laparoscopy.

Laparoscopic uterine nerve ablation by itself does not reduce endometriosis-associated pain.

Ablation of endometriotic lesions plus laparoscopic uterine nerve ablation (LUNA) in minimal-moderate disease reduces endometriosis associated pain.

There are no data supporting the use of uterine suspension but, in certain cases, there may be a role for presacral neurectomy especially in severe dysmenorrhea.

Ovarian Endometrioma

Superficial ovarian lesions can be coagulated or vaporized. The primary indication for extirpation of an endometrioma is to ensure it is not malignant. Small ovarian endometrioma (< 3 cm diameter) can be aspirated, irrigated, and inspected for intracystic lesions. Their interior wall can be coagulated or vaporized to destroy the mucosal lining. Ovarian endometriomas > 3 cm should be removed completely. Based on the current evidence, ovarian cystectomy seems to be the method of choice with a significantly decreased risk of cyst recurrence.

Moderate to Severe Degree of Endometriosis

If the endometriosis-related adhesions are part of an inflammatory fibrosis, they should be removed carefully. Radical procedures such as oophorectomy or total hysterectomy are indicted only in severe cases. If a hysterectomy is performed, the cervix should be extirpated as persistent pain in a remaining cervix is common due to endometriosis in the cervix or endometriosis in the uterosacral ligaments.

In a prospective, controlled, randomized, double-blind study, surgical therapy has been shown to be superior to expectant management six months after treatment of mild and moderate endometriosis. Treatment was least effective in women with minimal disease. One year later, symptom relief was still present in 90% of those who initially responded.

Although hormonal therapy prior to surgery improves rAFS scores, there is insufficient evidence of any effect on outcome measures such as pain relief.

Compared to surgery alone or surgery plus placebo, postoperative hormonal treatment does not produce a significant reduction in pain recurrence at 12 or 24 months, and has no effect on disease recurrence.

The ideal regimen for HRT after bilateral oophorectomy is unclear and should be discussed on an individual basis.

➲ TREATMENT OF ENDOMETRIOSIS RELATED SUBFERTILITY

Suppression of ovarian function to improve fertility in minimal–mild endo-metriosis is not effective and should not be offered for this indication alone. There is no evidence of its effectiveness in more severe disease.

Ablation of endometriotic lesions plus adhesiolysis to improve fertility in minimal–mild endometriosis is effective compared with diagnostic laparoscopy alone.

There is good evidence that excisional surgery for endometriomata provides for a more favorable outcome than drainage and ablation with regard to the recurrence of the endometrioma, recurrence of pain symptoms, and in women who were previously subfertile, subsequent spontaneous pregnancy. Consequently, this approach should be the favored surgical approach. However in women who may subsequently may undergo fertility treatment insufficient evidence exists to determine the favored surgical approach.

Excisional cystectomy is the preferred method to treat endometrial cysts for both pain and fertility and may be aided by the use of mesna and initial circular excision. An absorbable adhesion barrier (Interceed), 4% icodextrin solution (Adept), and a viscoelastic gel (Oxiplex/AP, FzioMed Inc, San Luis Obispd, CA; not available in the United States) are safe and effective products to help prevent adhesions in laparoscopic surgery to treat endometriosis.

Laparoscopic cystectomy for ovarian endometriomas is better than drainage and coagulation.

Ovarian reserve determined by AMH is less diminished after the three-step procedure compared with cystectomy of endometriomas.

No RCTs or meta-analyses are available to answer the question whether surgical excision of moderate to severe endometriosis enhances pregnancy rate.

Tubal flushing with oil-soluble media in infertile women is associated with a significant increase in clinical pregnancy rates. The effect is most pronounced in women with endometriosis.

➲ ASSISTED REPRODUCTION IN ENDOMETRIOSIS

Treatment with intrauterine insemination (IUI) improves fertility in minimal-mild endometriosis: IUI with ovarian stimulation is effective but the role of unstimulated IUI is uncertain.

In vitro fertilization (IVF) is appropriate treatment especially if tubal function is compromised, if there is also male factor infertility, and/or other treatments have failed. IVF pregnancy rates are lower in patients with endometriosis than in those with tubal infertility.

Treatment with a GnRH agonist for 3 to 6 months before IVF or ICSI should be considered in women with endometriosis as it increases the odds of clinical pregnancy fourfold. However, the authors of the Cochrane review stressed that the recommendation is based on only one properly randomized study and called for further research, particularly on the mechanism of action.

Controlled ovarian hyperstimulation (COH) for IVF/ICSI is equally effective with both GnRH antagonist and GnRH-aprotocols in terms of implantation and clinical pregnancy rates, but COH with GnRHa may be preferred because of the availability of more MII oocytes and embryos.

Risk for recurrence is no reason to withhold IVF therapy after surgery for endometriosis stage III or IV since cumulative endometriosis recurrence rates are not increased after ovarian hyperstimulation for IVF.

Laparoscopic ovarian cystectomy in patients with unilateral endometriomas between 3 and 6 cm in diameter before IVF/ICSI can decrease ovarian response without improving cycle outcome.

Overall, laparoscopic surgical removal of ovarian endometriotic cysts prior to IVF does not offer any additional benefit in terms of fertility outcomes. We thus recommend generally proceeding directly to IVF to reduce time to pregnancy, to avoid potential surgical complications and to limit patient costs. Surgery should be envisaged in specific circumstances, such as to treat concomitant pain symptoms which are refractory to medical treatments, or when malignancy cannot be reliably ruled out, or in the presence of large cysts. The diameter threshold for performing an operation before IVF should be adjusted according to the endometrioma location within the ovary. All decisions to operate a cyst beyond 3 or 4 cm are arbitrary, as there is no evidence to support one or the other. Surgeons should bear in mind that if all healthy growing follicles may be reached without damaging the endometrioma, cyst over 4 or even 5 cm do not require surgery in asymptomatic patients; however, smaller cysts that hide growing follicles, specially when the ovary is fixed, may require intervention.

➲ EXTRA GENITAL ENDOMETRIOSIS

Endometriosis can be found in almost any tissue in the body apart from the spleen. Symptoms will depend on the site of the disease. Cyclicity of symptoms is usually present, at least in early stages, and may be the only clue which leads to the diagnosis of endometriosis. Treatment will again depend on the site.

Appendicular endometriosis is usually treated by appendectomy. Surgical treatment of bladder endometriosis is usually in the form of excision of the lesion and primary closure of the bladder wall. Ureteral lesions may be excised after stenting the ureter, however in the presence of intrinsic lesions or significant obstruction segmental excision with end-to-end anastomosis or reimplantation may be necessary.

Abdominal wall and perineal endometriosis is usually treated by complete excision of the nodule.

Endometriotic lesions of the pleura, lung parenchyma and the diaphragmatic surface may present with pneumothorax, hemothorax, hemoptysis, chest pain and dyspnea. The symptoms are in general cyclical and tend to start within 24 to 48 hours after the onset of menstruation. Endometriotic lesions of the pleura, lung parenchyma and the diaphragmatic surface may present with pneumothorax, hemothorax, hemoptysis, chest pain and dyspnea. The symptoms are in general cyclical and tend to start within 24 to 48 hours after the onset of menstruation.

➲ COMPLEMENTARY THERAPY

Given the chronic and stubborn nature of endometriosis, there may be times when it can be beneficial to extend the therapeutic network beyond the medical mainstream; especially when women report that nutritional and complementary therapies, such as homeopathy, reflexology, traditional Chinese medicine (TCM), herbal treatments, physiotherapy, etc. improve their pain symptoms.

Whilst there is little evidence from any of the above to support these treatments in endometriosis related symptoms these should not be ruled out if the woman feels that they are beneficial to her overall pain management and/or quality of life.

Nutritional Therapy/Dietary Modification

Nutritional therapy/dietary modification has shown promising effects on dysmenorrhea in three small RCTs, specifically supplementation with omega-3 fish oil combined with vitamin B_{12} and a diet high in vegetables and low in animal fats.

Intake of fruit and green vegetables decreased the risk of endometriosis, whereas ham, beef and other red meat increased the risk. Several studies also link fiber intake to an increased estrogen excretion.

A randomized comparative study evaluated conservative surgery plus placebo compared with conservative surgery plus hormonal suppression treatment or dietary therapy (vitamins, minerals, lactic ferments, fish oil). It showed that hormonal suppression therapy and dietary supplementation were equally effective in reducing nonmenstrual pelvic pain and improving quality of life compared with placebo in women with endometriosis stage III–IV An RCT of 80 women with endometriosis demonstrated that two months of high-dose vitamin E and C therapy was associated with significant improvement in endometriosis pain and a reduction in inflammatory markers.

Homeopathy

In a very small, nonrandomised, study in eight patients diagnosed with endometriosis, five out of seven, who had dysmenorrhea, reported relief from symptoms (and two had intermittent relief) following individualized homeopathic treatment.

Herbal Remedies/Traditional Chinese Medicine

A systematic review of clinical and experimental data on the use of medicinal herbs in the treatment of endometriosis suggest that medical botanicals may have anti-inflammatory and pain-alleviating properties. Medicinal herbs and their active components exhibit cytokine-suppressive, COX-2- inhibiting, antioxidant, sedative and pain-alleviating properties. Each of these mechanisms of action would be predicted to have salutary effects in endometriosis.

Furthermore, Qu et al have demonstrated in endometriosis model rats that the Chinese herb Yiweining (YWN) can prevent the growth of ectopic endometrium by inhibiting the synthesis and secretion of TNF-α, IL-6, and IL-8, and can reduce the positive expressions of MMP-2 and COX-2 mRNAs.

Exercise

Whereas physiotherapy, yoga, pilates, and gentle exercise may assist the body in getting back into shape during/after prolonged periods of pain and/or after surgery to strengthen compromised pelvic/abdominal/back muscles, and whereas reflexology has anecdotally been reported to relieve pain symptoms, there is no evidence published relating to their therapeutic effect on dysmenorrhea or endometriosis-related symptoms.

Coaching and self-management programs may prove beneficial in providing the woman with tools to enable her to make informed decisions and learn to live with a chronic disease. Patient self-help groups can provide invaluable counseling, support and advice.

➲ REFERENCES

1. Al Kadri H, Hassan S, Al-Fozan HM, Hajeer A. Hormone therapy for endometriosis and surgical menopause. The Cochrane Library 2009;(1).
2. Birmingham, Alabama endometriosis and infertility. The Practice Committee of the American Society for Reproductive Medicine. Fertil Steril. 2006;86(4):S156–60.
3. Birmingham, Alabama treatment of pelvic pain associated with endometriosis. The Practice Committee of the American Society for Reproductive Medicine. Fertil Steril. 2008;90:S260–9.
4. Byung Chul Jee, Joong Yeup Lee, Chang Suk Suh, Seok Hyun Kim, Young Min Choi and Shin Yong Moon. Impact of GnRH agonist treatment on recurrence of ovarian endometriomas after conservative laparoscopic surgery. Fertil Steril 2009;91:40–5
5. Campos Petean C, Ferriani RA, Dos Reis RM, Dias de Moura M, Jordão AA Jr, Andrea de Albuquerque SNP. Lipid peroxidation and vitamin E in serum and follicular fluid of infertile women with peritoneal endometriosis submitted to controlled ovarian hyperstimulation: a pilot study. Fertil Steril. 2008.
6. Chul Jee B, et al. Impact of GnRH agonist treatment on recurrence of ovarian endometriomas after conservative laparoscopic surgery. Fertil Steril. 2009;91:40–5.
7. Coulter A, Ellins J. Effectiveness of strategies for informing, educating and involving patients. BMJ. 2007;335:24-7.
8. Daniel TR, Torsten S, Gerd B, Monika H, Ines MB, Arasen AVP, David TC and Martina B. Treatment of endometriosis with a VEGF-targeted conditionally replicative adenovirus. Fertil Steril. 2010; 93:2687–94.
9. Davis L, et al. "Modern combined oral contraceptives for pain associated with endometriosis." Cochrane Database Syst. Rev.3, 2007: CD001019.
10. Dimitrios T, George P, Dimitrios V, Dimitrios A, Tryfon T, Anastasia G and Basil CT. The impact on ovarian reserve after laparoscopic ovarian cystectomy versus three-stage management in patients with endometriomas: a prospective randomized study. Fertil Steril. 2010;94:71–7.
11. Edgardo S, Raffaella D, Paolo V, Giussy B, Laura B and Pier GC. The use and effectiveness of in vitro fertilization in women with endometriosis: the surgeon's perspective. Fertil Steril. 2009;91:1775–9.
12. Fjerbaek A and Knudsen UB. Endometriosis, dysmenorrhea and diet—what is the evidence? Eur J Obstet Gynecol Reprod Biol. 2007;132(2):140-7.
13. Flower A, Liu JP, Chen S, Lewith G, Little P. Chinese herbal medicine foe endometriosis. Cochrane Database Syst Rev. 2009.
14. Garcia-Velaso JA, Majutte NG, Corona J, Zuniga V, Giles J, Arici A, et al. Removal of endometriomas before in vitro fertilization does not improve fertility outcomes: a matched, case-control study. Fertil Steril. 2004;81:1194–7.
15. Geetu P, Tommaso F. Laparoscopic surgery for endometriosis-associated infertility: a pathophysiologic approach. Gynecol Surg. 2010. DOI 10.1007/s10397-010-0564-5.
16. Gomes MK, et al. "The levonorgestrel-releasing intrauterine system and endometriosis staging." Fertil Steril. 2007;87(5):1231-4.
17. Green-top Guideline No. 24. Oct 2006; RCOG.
18. Harada T, et al. "Low-dose oral contraceptive pill for dysmenorrhea associated with endometriosis: A placebo-controlled, double-blind, randomized trial." Fertil Steril. 2007.

19. Harada T, Momoeda A, Taketani B, Hoshiai B, Naoki Terakawa C. Low-dose oral contraceptive pill for dysmenorrhea associated with endometriosis: a placebo-controlled, double-blind, randomized trial. Fertil Steril. 2008;90:1583–8.

20. Hughes E, Brown J, Collins JJ, Farquhar C, Fedorkow DM, Vanderkerchove P. Ovulation suppression for endometriosis for women with subfertility. (Review) The Cochrane Library. 2010;(1).

21. Ioanna T, Maria K, Tarek AG and Luciano GN. The effect of surgical treatment for endometrioma on in vitro fertilization outcomes: a systematic review and meta-analysis. Fertil Steril. 2009;92:75–87.

22. Jacobson TZ, Duffy JMN, Barlow D, Farquhar C, Koninckx PR, Olive D. Laparoscopic surgery for subfertility associated with endometriosis. (Review) The Cochrane Library. 2010;(1).

23. Jacques D, Jean-Christophe L, Pascale J, Olivier D and Jean S. Laparoscopic management of endometriomas using a combined technique of excisional (cystectomy) and ablative surgery. Fertil Steril. 2010;94:28–32.

24. Juan A Garcia-Velasco, Somigliana E. Management of endometriomas in women requiring IVF: to touch or not to touch. Hum Reprod. 2009;1(1):1–6.

25. Kelly NW and Marc RL. Endometriomas in adolescents. Fertil Steril. 2010;94:1529. e7–e9.

26. Kennedy AD, Sculpher MJ, Coulter A, Dwyer N, Rees M, Abrams KR, et al. Effects of decision aids formenorrhagia on treatment choices, health outcomes, and costs: a randomized controlled trial. JAMA. 2002;288:2701-8.

27. Lian F, Liu HP, Wang YX, Zhang JW, Sun ZG, Ma FM, et al. Expressions of VEGF and Ki-67 in eutopic endometrium of patients with endometriosis and effect of Quyu Jiedu Recipe on VEGF expression. Chin J Integr Med. 2007;13(2):109-14.

28. Manheimer E, Zhang G, Udoff L, Haramati A, Landenberg P, Berman BM, et al.

29. Effects of acupuncture on rates of pregnancy and live birth among women undergoing in vitro fertilisation: systematic review and meta-analysis. BMJ 2008; 336:545-9.

30. Pabuccu R, Onalan A, Kaya C. GnRH agonist and antagonist protocols for stage I–II endometriosis and endometrioma in in vitro fertilization/ intracytoplasmic sperm injection cycles. Fertil Steril. 2007;88:832–9.

31. Paolo Vercellini, Edgardo omigliana, Paola Vigano, Annalisa Abbiati, Giussy Barbara and Pier Giorgio Crosignani. Surgery for endometriosis-associated infertility: a pragmatic approach. Hum Reprod. 2009;24(2): 254–69.

32. Patrick Y Jr., Ken S, Wendy W, Robert B Albee. Complete laparoscopic excision of endometriosis in teenagers: is postoperative hormonal suppression necessary? Fertil Steril. 2011;95:1909–12.

33. Razzi S, et al. "Efficacy of vaginal danazol treatment in women with recurrent deeply infiltrating endometriosis." Fertil Steril. 2007;88(4):789-94.

34. Remorgida V, et al. "Letrozole and desogestrel-only contraceptive pill for the treatment of stage IV endometriosis." Aust.N.Z.J Obstet.Gynaecol. 2007;47(3): 222-5.

35. Remorgida V, et al. "Letrozole and norethisterone acetate in rectovaginal endometriosis." Fertil Steril. 2007;88(3):724-6.

36. Renato S, Mohamed M, Giulia M, Linda M, Sergio C and Stefano V. Conservative laparoscopic management of urinary tract endometriosis (UTE): surgical outcome and long-term follow-up. Fertil Steril. 2010;94:856–61.

37. Sallam HN, Garcia-Velasco JA, Dias S, Arici A. Long-term pituitary down-regulation before in vitro fertilization (IVF) for women with endometriosis. (Review) The Cochrane Library. 2009;(1).

38. Sesti F, Pietropolli A, Capozzolo A, Broccoli A, Pierangeli A, Bollea B and Emilio P. Hormonal suppression treatment or dietary therapy versus placebo in the control of painful symptoms after conservative surgery for endometriosis stage III–IV. A randomized comparative trial. Fertil Steril. 2007; 88:1541–7.

39. Sesti F, Pietropolli A, Capozzolo T, Broccoli P, Pierangeli S, Bollea MR, et al. Hormonal suppression treatment or dietary therapy versus placebo in the control of painful symptoms after conservative surgery for endometriosis stage III–IV. A randomized comparative trial. Fertil Steril. 2007; 88(6):1541-7.

40. The ESHRE guideline on endometriosis, 2008.

41. The Practice Committee of the American Society for Reproductive Medicine. Endometriosis and infertility. Fertil Steril. 2004;81:1441–6.

42. Vercellini P, Crosignani, Abbiati A, Somigliana E, Vigano P and Fedele L. The effect of surgery for symptomatic endometriosis: the other side of the story. Hum Reprod Update, 2009;15(2): 177–188.

43. Wieser F, Cohen M, Gaeddert A, Jie Yu, Burks-Wicks C, Sarah L. Berga, et al. Evolution of medical treatment for endometriosis: back to the roots? Human Reproduction Update. 2007;3(5):487–99.

44. Wieser F, Cohen M, Gaeddert A, Yu J, Burks-Wicks C, Berga SL, et al. Evolution of medical treatment for endometriosis: back to the roots? Hum Reprod Update 2007;13(5):487-99.

Endometriosis: Future Thoughts

◀ Parul J Kotdawala, Sonal Kotdawala

Endometriosis has still remained an enigma for all of us. The disease has increased its prevalence overtime and has defied all attempts at unraveling the mystery about its origin, progression and its impact on a woman's reproductive life. Epidemiological studies estimate a prevalence of 6 to 10%, and it may be much higher if milder forms of the disease, which are underdiagnosed, are included. Many women have been rendered infertile and many more have led a painful life afflicted by this pervasive and insidious disease. The problem is not only its detection, which requires a laparoscopy—an invasive procedure—but the therapy is equally frustrating and fascinating for all of us who deal with this amazing disease.

As our current knowledge about this disease guides us, we have reached following consensus in dealing with women suffering with endometriosis;

1. The accurate diagnosis is made with laparoscopy, unless there is an endometriotic cyst (detected on ultrasonography) or when there is a visible vaginal nodule on inspection.
2. Laparoscopy is 'Gold Standard' diagnostic procedure for all forms of endometriosis.
3. A visual inspection of the lesion is adequate for a diagnosis of endo-. metriosis, but histological confirmation of at least one lesion is ideal.
4. Positive histology confirms the diagnosis, but negative does not exclude it
5. Histological examination fails to detect endometrium in about 50% of visible endometriosis.
6. Medical therapy alone has no role in women desirous of childbearing.
7. Medical therapy is a useful option for women desirous of pain relief only.
8. All medical therapy like COC, progesterones, danazol, GnRHA have almost similar efficacy.
9. When the patient is given antiestrogen therapy (e.g. progesterones, GnRHa) it should be covered with calcium and vitamin D to prevent osteoporosis.
10. Medical therapy is not effective in pain symptom of rectovaginal endo-metriosis and removal of rectovaginal nodule is necessary for alleviation of pain symptoms.
11. Destruction or excision of endometriotic implants in all stages and all forms of disease improves pregnancy outcomes as well as reduces pain.

12. In case of endometriotic cyst a cystectomy reduces the chances of recurrence and improves chances of pregnancy.
13. There is still a lack of clarity about the optimum role of medical therapy before or after the surgery for endometriosis.

Upon this background, I am trying to share with you some exciting and promising developments taking place in diagnosis as well as in the therapy of endometriosis.

⊃ DIAGNOSIS OF ENDOMETRIOSIS

As we all know, the only reliable and accurate method of diagnosis is by visual inspection of peritoneal cavity and locating the lesion or a histopathological confirmation of a biopsy obtained at a laparoscopy (or a laparotomy). Naturally, the procedure is not a first line diagnostic tool. As it requires anesthesia and as the procedure has significant morbidity—both, the patients as well as the doctors are reluctant to undertake the procedure quickly. This has led to a delay of average 9 years in diagnosis.

A recent survey among 7025 women respondents with endometriosis (European Endometriosis Alliance, 2006) demonstrated that 65% of the women with endometriosis were first misdiagnosed with another condition, and 46% had to see five doctors or more before they were correctly diagnosed, resulting in an average delay of 8 years between the onset of symptoms and the diagnosis of endometriosis (Zondervan et al 1999; Ballard et al 2006).

Currently used non-invasive approaches for the diagnosis like USG, MRI or blood tests (CA-125) have not been accurate enough for the diagnosis of endometriosis. (Chen et al 1998; Zondervan et al 1999; Harada et al 2002; Somigliana et al 2004; Kennedy et al 2005; Ballard et al 2006, Mol et al 1998).

A subfertile woman with a history of menstrual pain and normal clinical examination in absence of positive USG for endometriotic cysts provides a dilemma for most gynecologists. The advice for a laparoscopy is not confident enough and patient's reluctance for invasive procedure in absence of firm recommendation delays the diagnosis. From a clinical perspective, it is unlikely that these women will have moderate-to-severe endometriosis, but up to 50% of them (Meuleman et al 2009) may have mild peritoneal endometriosis with or without adhesions associated with subfertility and possibly pain. A non-invasive diagnostic test would be useful to rule out endometriosis in this group of women and may benefit them for a more precise management of subfertility therapy (D'Hooghe et al 2003, 2006; Kennedy et al 2005).

With this limitation in mind there has been extensive research for a simpler diagnostic tool and few papers published recently have shown great promise. Two main evolving methods of diagnosis are biochemical methods and histological evaluation of uterine endometrium.

Biochemical Methods

A recent study published in Human Reproduction (Mihalyi, Gevaert et al 2009, 2010) has shown great promise in making accurate diagnosis of endometriosis. The study involves a combined analysis of 6 biomarkers using stepwise logistic regression analysis and least squares support vector machines (LSSVMs). The study shows that it is possible to diagnose minimal–mild endometriosis using plasma analysis of multiple biomarkers combined with advanced statistical analysis with a high sensitivity (87 to 92%) and an acceptable specificity (60 to 71%) during the secretory phase and the menstrual phase.

This case–control study was conducted in 294 infertile women, consisting of 93 women with a normal pelvis and 201 women with endometriosis. They measured plasma concentrations of:
1. Interleukin IL-6 (0.71 vs 0.34 pg/ml)
2. Interleukin IL-8 (1.77 vs 0.88 pg/ml)
3. Cancer antigen CA 125 (22.0 vs 13.0 U/ml)
4. Cancer antigen CA 19-9
5. Tumor necrosis factor-α (TNF-α) (0.03 vs 0.44 pg/ml)
6. High-sensitivity C-reactive protein (hsCRP) (1.35 vs 0.64 mg/l).

Compared with controls, both women with minimal–mild and moderate–severe endometriosis had higher plasma levels of IL-6, IL-8 and CA-125 and lower levels of TNF-α regardless of cycle phase. In addition, women with moderate–severe endometriosis had significantly higher hsCRP levels than controls Using stepwise logistic regression, moderate–severe endometriosis was diagnosed with a sensitivity of 100% (specificity 84%) during the secretory phase. Using LSSVM analysis, minimal–mild endometriosis was diagnosed with a sensitivity of 94% (specificity 61%) during the secretory phase and during the menstrual phase.

Another study published (Gajbhiye, Sonawani et al 2011) very recently use a proteomic approach to identify novel endometrial antigens using sera from endometriosis patients and healthy controls, with evaluation of biomarkers for non invasive diagnosis of endometriosis. They conducted a cross-sectional study to identify specific endometrial antigens in women with early endometriosis (n = 17), advanced endometriosis (n = 23) and without endometriosis (n = 30). The study identified 3 endometrial antigens; tropomyosin 3 (TPM3), stomatin-like protein 2 (SLP2), and tropomodulin 3 (TMOD3). Serum levels of antibodies against the proteins TPM3, SLP2 and TMOD3 were significantly elevated in endometriosis patients when compared with controls. The sensitivity and specificity of serum antibodies were calculated to:
❖ Anti-TPM3a-Ab (61%, 93%), anti-TPM3c-Ab (44%, 93%), anti-TPM3d-Ab (78%, 89%)
❖ Anti-SLP2a-Ab (50%, 96%), anti-SLP2c-Ab (61%, 93%)
❖ Anti-TMOD3b-Ab (61%, 96%), anti-TMOD3c-Ab (78%, 93%), anti-TMOD3d-Ab (78%, 96%)

The authors concluded that serum levels of antibodies against the proteins TPM3, SLP2 and TMOD3 were better than those of serum CA125 levels (21%, 89%) in the detection of early stages of endometriosis. The high specificity shown in this study (90% + in all markers) suggest that the accuracy is of high order and the false negative diagnosis will be very low.

I believe that we are on threshold of an accurate and useful blood test to make an easy and early diagnosis of endometriosis. This will be a great step forward in managing this curious scourge of women. These tests sound familiar in the connotation of 'six markers' and 'three markers'.

Endometrial Histology

In the search for a non-invasive diagnostic test scientists have found multiple-sensory small-diameter nerve fibers in a higher density in endometrium from patients with endometriosis compared to women with a normal pelvis. This fact has enabled a development of a semi-invasive diagnostic test for minimal–mild endometriosis.

In a classical study titled 'Density of small diameter sensory nerve fibers in endometrium: a semi-invasive diagnostic test for minimal to mild endometriosis' published in Human Reproduction, (Bokor, Kyama et al) from University of Leuven, Belgium collected secretory phase endometrium samples (n 40), obtained from women with laparoscopically/ histologically confirmed minimal-mild endometriosis (n 20) and from women with a normal pelvis (n 20). Immunohistochemistry was performed to localize neural markers for sensory nerve fibers in the functional layer of the endometrium. Sections were immunostained with antihuman protein gene product 9.5 (PGP 9.5), anti-neurofilament protein, antisubstance P (SP), antivasoactive intestinal peptide (VIP), antineuropeptide Y and anticalcitonine gene-related polypeptide. The density of small nerve fibers was approximately 14 times higher in endometrium from patients with minimal-mild endometriosis (1.96 +/– 2.73) when compared with women with a normal pelvis (0.14 +/– 0.46). The combined analysis of neural markers PGP9.5, VIP and SP could predict the presence of minimal-mild endometriosis with 95% sensitivity, 100% specificity and 97.5% accuracy.

Another prospective and equally classical study 'Diagnosis of endometriosis by detection of nerve fibers in an endometrial biopsy: a double blind study' published in Human Reproduction by (Al-Jefout, Dezarnaulds et al) showed in a double blind comparison with expert diagnostic laparoscopy a high presence of nerve fibers in endometrium. Endometrial biopsies, with immunohistochemical nerve fiber detection using protein gene product 9.5 as marker, taken from 99 consecutive women presenting with pelvic pain and/ or infertility undergoing diagnostic laparoscopy by experienced gynecologic laparoscopists, were compared with surgical diagnosis.

In women with laparoscopic diagnosis of endometriosis (n 64) the mean nerve fiber density in the functional layer of the endometrial biopsy was 2.7

nerve fibers/mm^2. Only one woman with endometriosis had no detectable nerve fibers. Six women had endometrial nerve fibers but no active endometriosis seen at laparoscopy. The specificity and sensitivity were 83 and 98%, respectively, positive predictive value was 91% and negative predictive value was 96%. Nerve fiber density did not differ between different menstrual cycle phases. Women with endometriosis and pain symptoms had significantly higher nerve fiber density in comparison with women with infertility but no pain (2.3 and 0.8 nerve fiber/mm^2, respectively).

This study clearly shows that an endometrial biopsy, with detection of nerve fibers, provides a reliability of diagnosis of endometriosis which is close to the accuracy of laparoscopic assessment. Although semi-invasive in nature it obviates all the complications attached to a laparoscopy.

⤳ THERAPY FOR ENDOMETRIOSIS

Although there is a loose consensus on therapeutic principles for both, pain and infertility associated with endometriosis, I would like to share some fresh developments which chart a new course.

Antiestrogen Therapies: COC, Progesterones, Danazol, Gestrinone

Suppression of ovarian hormones to induce amenorrhea is the basis for most medical treatments in endometriosis. Combined OC pills (COC) with estrogen and progesterone combination (E+P) suppress ovarian folliculogenesis and steroid secretion, and induce amenorrhea of so-called pseudopregnancy in the management of endometriosis. Progestogens alone have a similar though less consistent effect. Due to a direct stimulatory effect on the endometriotic tissue E+P is often suboptimal in providing symptom relief if dysmenoorrhea is the major complaint. Danazol was the first compound that could effectively suppress ovarian function without a direct effect on the endometrium. One of the interesting properties of danazol is its effect on the immune system. However, its androgenic side effects made it less attractive to patients and physicians. Danazol vaginal delivery systems and danazol-releasing IUD are under development in a bid to avert the systemic side effects. LNG–IUD ('Mirena'), once a week COC skin patch and the COC vaginal ring are also tried for long-term pain relief in endometriosis to avoid the systemic side effects.

Gonadotropin-Releasing Hormone Agonists (GnRHa)

This has been one of the most effective and popular option in the postoperative treatment of endometriosis. These compounds profoundly suppress ovarian function and induce endometrial atrophy and amenorrhea after the initial stimulatory flare up effect. Agonists are currently available only for parenteral use as depot imtramuscular (IM) injections, subcutaneous depot implants/injections, or intranasal sprays. The daily release dose of agonist is adjusted in such a way that complete pituitary suppression is induced. FSH and LH levels are undetectable and estradiol remains < 20 pg/ml. This profound ovarian suppression results in amenorrhea, symptomatic improvement, and regression of endometriotic lesions. However, at the same time a majority of women develop menopausal symptoms, hypoestrogenic changes, and bone loss. In order to reduce the severity of menopausal symptoms and to prevent bone loss, various estrogen/progestogen add-back regimens have been recommended.

It has been theorized by (Barbieri 1998) that estradiol levels between 30 to 50 pg/ml are effective in inducing endometrial atrophy but the levels leading to bone loss is much lower (< 20 pg). Thus, a therapeutic window of estradiol levels adequate for suppression of endometriosis without untoward side effects is available.

Agonists are not suitable in patients with PCO due to its inconsistent suppressive effect and have significant side effect profile during the initial flare-up. Peptide Gonadotropin-releasing hormone antagonists structurally resemble native GnRH and GnRH agonists. Unlike agonists, antagonists competitively block GnRH receptors and produce an immediate suppressive effect on the pituitary, leading to quick reduction in serum FSH and LH levels. GnRH antagonists had troublesome side effects like injection-site reactions and allergic/anaphylactic reactions related to histamine release from mast cells. Cetrorelix, a peptide GnRH antagonist, is approved for suppression of LH surge in women undergoing *in vitro* fertilization (IVF). In clinical trials cetrorelix was found effective in controlling pelvic pain and in inducing regression of endometriosis on post-treatment laparoscopy (Finas, Hornung et al 2006). The effect was immediate, without flare-up, and the course of treatment was shorter than that with GnRH agonists.

Peptide GnRH analogs, both agonists and antagonists, require parenteral administration in the form of long-acting depots. This is associated with prolonged effect and inability to rapidly terminate the treatment when necessary. Recently several non-peptide small-molecule GnRH antagonists have been developed which are orally active. This improves patient acceptability, facilitates dosing and allows rapid discontinuation if necessary. We can also plan dose adjustment to vary the level of pituitary suppression and the circulating estradiol levels in the therapeutic window. This may facilitate long-term treatment without the need for addback therapy.

Oral GnRH Antagonists

Elagolix (NBI-56418) is a small non-peptide GnRH Antagonist molecule that binds reversibly with high affinity to the human GnRH receptor. Elagolix has recently completed phase II clinical trials in women with pelvic pain associated with endometriosis. The drug is rapidly absorbed from the GI tract, reach maximum plasma concentration within 30 to 60 minutes after ingestion, followed by a rapid decline in blood levels. Elagolix induces dose-dependent FSH, LH, and estradiol suppression without detectable flare effect. At a dose of

100 to 150 mg/day, serum estradiol concentrations remained between 20 to 50 pg/ml, which seems to be the optimal range (Dmowski 2008. Struthers et al 2009).

Elagolix seems to be well-tolerated in comparison with placebo. The most common side effects reported were headaches, nausea, and dizziness. The reporting of hot flashes with doses ranging from 50 to 200 mg was 49.3% compared with 42.6% in the placebo groups. None of the women receiving elagolix reported severe vasomotor or hypoestrogenic symptoms. There was no increase in serum N-telopeptide concentrations, a biomarker for bone resorption. There was improvement in the composite pelvic signs and symptoms score (CPSSS) and the visual analog scale (VAS) for pelvic pain scores, which was most pronounced at doses of 150 mg once daily and 100 mg twice daily. Return of regular ovulatory cycles, as evidenced by urinary pregnanediol measurements, was rapid in most patients. Availability of oral therapy which can be titrated to individual needs is one of the most exciting developments in the field of endometriosis management.

Diet, Habitus and Alternative Therapies

There are by now adequate studies to establish relationship between diet, body habitus, mental stress and endometriosis. Alternative therapies become an attractive option under these situations. Various forms of nutritional therapy, dietary modifications, exercise plans, homeopathy medicines and immune therapy have been proposed with observational reports.

Lending credence to the current fad of lean figure and increasing incidence of endometriosis in young adolescents, in a very interesting study published recently, women diagnosed with endometriosis were taller, thinner, and had a significantly lower BMI. They were late maturers (menarche $\geq$ 14 years) and late to initiate sexual activity ($\geq$ 21 years.) For every unit increase in BMI (kg/m^2), there was an approximate 12 to 14% decrease in the likelihood of being diagnosed with endometriosis. BMI was 21.3 for women with endometriosis, compared with 23.2 for the controls, a difference over all ages of –1.9. This is a consistent difference of about 10 lb at every age, assuming an average height of about 64.5 in. The authors concluded that women diagnosed with endometriosis may have a consistently lean physique during adolescence and young adulthood with a supposition that there might be an *in utero* or early childhood origin for endometriosis (Hediger et al 2005).

Chinese Herbal Medicines (CHM)

A recent Cochrane review on Chinese herbal medicines has shown promising results. Two Chinese RCTs involving 158 women were included in this review. Both these trials described adequate methodology.

CHM vs Gestrinone

There was no evidence of a significant difference in rates of symptomatic relief between CHM and gestrinone administered subsequent to laparoscopic surgery (95.65% vs 93.87%). The intention-to-treat analysis also showed no significant difference between the groups. There was no significant difference between the CHM and gestrinone groups with regard to the total pregnancy rate (69.6% vs 59.1%, one RCT).

CHM vs Danazol

CHM was administered orally and then in conjunction with a herbal enema resulted in a greater proportion of women obtaining symptomatic relief than with danazol. Overall, 100% of women in all the groups showed some improvement in their symptoms. Oral plus enema administration of CHM showed a greater reduction in average dysmenorrhea pain scores than did danazol. Combined oral and enema administration of CHM showed a greater improvement, measured as the disappearance or shrinkage of adnexal masses, than with danazol. For lumbosacral pain, rectal discomfort, or vaginal nodules tenderness, there was no significant difference either between CHM and danazol.

The authors went on to conclude that postsurgical administration of CHM may have comparable benefits to gestrinone but with fewer side effects. Oral CHM may have a better overall treatment effect than danazol; it may be more effective in relieving dysmenorrhea and shrinking adnexal masses when used in conjunction with a CHM enema. However, more rigorous research may confirm the potential role of CHM in treating endometriosis (Flower et al 2009).

Aromatase Inhibitors

An interesting publication (Ailawadi, Bulun et al 2004) showed marked benefits of Latrozole in clearing up endometriosis within 6 months of therapy in cases with pain. Letrozole 2.5 mg + progestin 2.5 mg + vitamin D 800 IU + calcium 1.25 gm were given for 6 months and a 2nd look laparoscopy and biopsy was performed. In all cases the endometriosis disappeared! A few subsequent studies have also confirmed these findings. Aromataze enzymes are found in 3 places; ovaries, adipose tissues and endometriotic implants. Conventional therapy (GnRH agonists, danazol, progestins) suppresses the ovarian tissues, but do not have a major effect on other tissues, and hence their effects are transitory. Aromataze inhibitors suppress all three locations and hence their superiority.

Aromatase P450 is the key enzyme for estrogen biosynthesis, catalyzing the conversion of androstenedione and testosterone to estrone and estradiol. Although the normal endometrium contains no detectable levels of aromatase activity, this enzyme is active with high levels in endometriotic tissue and increase local estrogen production. Aromatase inhibitors target this enzyme to decrease local estrogen synthesis and thus to inhibit the growth of endometriotic implants. However, this treatment also would reduce ovarian estrogen production and may therefore require estrogen add-back therapy to protect bones. This usage should be limited to the small number of severe cases of women with pelvic endometriosis causing intractable pain. Long-term therapy should of course be monitored with bone density scans and low-dose add-back hormone replacement therapy (HRT). We can offer very little, other than radical pelvic surgery with its potential risks, to a women with intractable endometriosis related pelvic pain. Aromatase inhibitor therapy may be justified in these cases, despite a limited evidence base.

Lipiodol Flushing

An interesting study published in 'Fertility Society of Australia, Neil Jhonson, University of Aukland, Nov 2003' used the oil based dye to flush the fallopian tubes as done at HSG. This flushes out debris from tubes that is not actually blocking but which in some ways is hindering pregnancy. This also reduces the stickiness of fimbria and in some way reduces the embryotoxicity of tubal milieu. The study was carried out on 158 patients with 5+ years of infertility, and there was 4.5 times rise in pregnancy rate over next 6 months.

Photodynamic Therapy (PDT)

Photodynamic therapy is based on the selective destruction of growing tissue resulting from interaction between photosensitizer, light and oxygen. Primarily used in cancer cases this therapy has shown great initial potential. In last decade, there have been 20+ publications about the use of this technology for endometriosis treatment.

SERMs and SPRMs

Selective Estrogen Receptor Modulators are dubbed "designer estrogens" because they mimic the action of estrogen where it's wanted, such as in the cardiovascular and skeletal systems, but avoid estrogenic action where it's not; i.e. breast and uterine tissue. SERMs have been shown in animal studies to prevent bone loss and estrogenic proliferation; In one study on rhesus monkeys with endometriosis, treatment with SERMs resulted in decreased uterine size and significant decreases in lesion size. There are several SERM studies underway, including one at the National Institutes of Health on the use of raloxifine in patients with endometriosis.

Terbutaline

Currently used to prevent premature labor, studies are underway to determine the efficacy of this drug as potential treatment for endometriosis pain. Terbutaline relaxes the uterine muscles and can be helpful in easing menstrual pain related to the disease.

Mifepristone (RU-486)

The controversial so-called abortion drug may have implications in treating endometriosis. RU-486, an anti-progestin, binds itself to progesterone receptors on the wall of the uterus and blocks the effect of the woman's natural progesterone. In addition to its antiprogestin and antiglucocoritcoid properties, RU-486 is also a noncompetitive antiestrogen. As such, RU-486 blocks the capacity of the endometrial tissue to grow in response to estrogen, making mifepristone a possible hormonal treatment for endometriosis.

Angiogenesis (Stopping the Lesion at its Source)

Angiogenesis holds that ectopic tissue requires blood supply, regardless of size, location or theory of implantation. Without blood vessel development, hormone impact can be negated. Hence, endometriosis lesions can be potentially destroyed by cutting off their blood supply. Angiogenesis has interesting implications on the prevention of adhesion formation as well. It may be shown through further studies that this highly complex and unique technique holds real opportunity for treatment in endometriosis, whether alone or as an adjunct therapy.

Endocrine Disrupters

Cleaning up our act (and our environment), dioxins are one such pollutant.

Endocrine disrupters are chemicals present in our environment that, by virtue of their ability to interact with the endocrine system, are causing a variety of adverse health effects in humans and animals. Because the endocrine system plays such a critical role in normal growth, development and reproduction, even small disturbances in function may have profound and lasting effects. (Rier S, Foster W 2002)

The US Environmental Protection Agency clearly describes dioxin as a serious public health threat. The EPA report states, there is no "safe" level of exposure to dioxin-even trace amounts are a risk. Further, the EPA report confirmed that "dioxin is a cancer hazard to people; that exposure to dioxin can also cause severe reproductive and developmental problems (at levels 100 times lower than those associated with its cancer causing effects); and that dioxin can cause immune system damage and interfere with regulatory hormones."

Evidence of dioxin as a catalyst for endometriosis has been well-documented. In a 1996 Environmental Protection Agency study, dioxin exposure was linked with increased risks for endometriosis, as well as the increased risks of pelvic inflammatory disease, reduction of fertility, and interference with normal fetal and childhood development. According to a February 2000 report from the Food and Drug Administration, tampons and feminine hygiene products currently sold in the US are made of cotton, rayon, or blends of rayon and cotton. Even though these products are now produced using elemental chlorine free or totally chlorine free bleaching processes, these methods can still generate dioxins at "trace levels." Thus, there may be low amounts of dioxin present from environmental sources in cotton, rayon, or rayon/cotton tampons and feminine hygiene products. Using safe products will go a long way in preventing endometriosis.

Iron Chelators

In a path breaking review titled 'Potential involvement of iron in the pathogenesis of peritoneal endometriosis', (Defre`re, Donnez et al) suggest that in endometriosis patients, iron overload has been demonstrated in the different components of the peritoneal cavity (peritoneal fluid, endometriotic lesions, peritoneum and macrophages). Animal models suggest that this may originate from erythrocytes carried into the pelvic cavity mainly by retrograde menstruation. Peritoneal macrophages play an important role in the degradation of these erythrocytes and in subsequent peritoneal iron metabolism. Iron overload could affect a wide range of mechanisms involved in endometriosis development, such as oxidative stress or lesion proliferation. They concluded that excess iron accumulation can result in toxicity and may be one of the factors contributing to the development of endometriosis. Treatment with an iron chelator could thus be beneficial in endometriosis patients to prevent iron overload in the pelvic cavity, thereby diminishing its deleterious effect.

⊃ REFERENCES

1. Ailawadi RK, Jobanputra S, Kataria M, Gurates B, Bulun SE. Treatment of endometriosis and chronic pelvic pain with letrozole and norethindrone acetate: a pilot study. Fertil Steril. 2004;81: 290–6.
2. Al-Jefout M, Dezarnaulds G, Cooper M, et al. Diagnosis of endometriosis by detection of nerve fibers in an endometrial biopsy: a double blind study. Human Reproduction. 2009;24(12):3019–24.
3. Ballard KD, Lowton K, Wright JT. What's the delay? A qualitative study of women's experience of reaching a diagnosis of endometriosis. Fertil Steril. 2006;85:1296-1301.
4. Barbieri RL. Endometriosis and the estrogen threshold theory in relation to surgical and medical treatment, J Reprod Med. 1998;43(Suppl. 3):287–92.
5. Billen J, Blanckaert N, Vodolazkaia A, Fulop V, D'Hooghe T M. Non-invasive diagnosis of endometriosis based on a combined analysis of six plasma biomarkers. Hum Reprod. 2009:1–11.
6. Bokor CM, Kyama L, Vercruysse et al. Density of small diameter sensory nerve fibers in endometrium: a semi-invasive diagnostic test for minimal to mild endometriosis. Hum Reprod. 2009;24(12):3025–32.
7. Bulun S, Fang Z, Imir G, Gurates B. Aromatase and endometriosis. Semin Reprod Med. 2004;22:45–50.
8. Chen FP, Soong YK, Lee N, Lo SK. The use of serum CA-125 as a marker for endometriosis in patients with dysmenorrhea for monitoring therapy and for recurrence of endometriosis. Acta Obstet Gynecol Scand. 1998;77:665-70.
9. D'Hooghe TM, Debrock S, Hill JA, Meuleman C. Endometriosis and subfertility: is the relationship resolved? Semin Reprod Med. 2003;21:243-54.
10. D'Hooghe TM, Mihalyi AM, Simsa P, Kyama CK, Peeraer K, De Loecker P, at al. Why we need a noninvasive diagnostic test for minimal to mild endometriosis with a high sensivity. Gynecol Obstet Invest. 2006;62:136-8.
11. Defre`re S, Lousse JC, Gonza´lez-Ramos R, Colette S, Donnez J , A Van Langendonckt. Potential involvement of iron in the pathogenesis of peritoneal endometriosis; Mol Hum Reprod. 2008;14(7):377–85.

12. Dmowski WP. Advances in the treatment of endometriosis—the potential of elagolix (NBI-56418). US Obste and Gynec. 2008;3(1):21-3.
13. European Endometriosis Alliance. Endometriosis. www.endometriosis.org, 2006.
14. Finas D, Hornung D, Diedrich K, Schultze-Mosgau A. Cetrorelix in the treatment of female infertility and endometriosis. Expert Opin Pharmacother. 2006;7(15):2155-68.
15. Flower A, Liu JP, Chen S, Lewith G, Little P. Chinese herbal medicine for endometriosis. Cochrane Database of Systematic Reviews. 2009;3. Art. No.: CD006568.
16. Food and Drug Administration, USA 2000.
17. Gajbhiye R, Sonawani A, Khan S, Suryawanshi A, Kadam S, Warty N, et al. Identification and validation of novel serum markers for early diagnosis of endometriosis, Hum. Reprod. 2011.
18. Hadfleld R, Mardon H, Barlow D, Kennedy S. Delay in the diagnosis of endometriosis: a survey of women from the USA and the UK. Hum Reprod. 1996;11(4):878-80.
19. Harada T, Kubota T, Aso T. Usefulness of CA19-9 versus CA125 for the diagnosis of endometriosis. Fertil Steril. 2002;78:733-9.
20. Hediger ML, Hartnett HJ, Buck Louis Germaine M. Association of endometriosis with body size and figure. Fertil Steril. 2005;84(5):1366–74.
21. Kaylon L, Bruner-Tran, Grant R, Yeaman, Marta A Crispens, Toshio M. Dioxin may promote inflammation-related development of endometriosis. Fertil Steril. 2008; 89 (5):1287–98.
22. Kennedy S, Bergqvist A, Chapron C, et al. ESHRE guideline for the diagnosis and treatment of endometriosis. Hum Reprod. 2005;20(10):2698-704.
23. Meuleman C, Vandenabeele B, Fieuws S, Spiessens C, Timmerman D, D'Hooghe T. High prevalence of endometriosis in infertile women with normal ovulation and normospermic partners. Fertil Steril. 2009;92(1):68-74.
24. Mihalyi A, Gevaert O, Kyama CM, Simsa P, Pochet N, De Smet F, et al. Non-invasive diagnosis of endometriosis based on a combined analysis of six plasma biomarkers; Human Reproduction. 2010;25(3):654–64.
25. Mihalyi O, Gevaert CM, Kyama P, Simsa N, Pochet F, De Smet B, et al. Non-invasive diagnosis of endometriosis based on a combined analysis of six plasma biomarkers Hum Reprod. 2010;25(3):654-64.
26. Mol BWJ, Bayram N, Lijmer JG et al. The performance of CA-125 measurement in the detection of endometriosis: a meta-analysis. Fertil Steril. 1998;70:1101.
27. Patwardhan S, Nawathe A, Yates D, Harrison G, Khan K. Systematic review of the effects of aromatase inhibitors on pain associated with endometriosis. BJOG. 2008;115:818–22.
28. Rier S, Warren GF. Environmental dioxins and endometriosis, toxicological sciences. 70(2):161-70.
29. Somigliana E, Vigano P, Tirelli AS, Felicetta I, Torresani E, Vignali M, et al. Use of the concomitant serum dosage of CA 125, CA 19-9 and interleukin-6 to detect the presence of endometriosis. Results from a series of reproductive age women undergoing laparoscopic surgery for benign gynaecological conditions. Hum Reprod. 2004;19:1871-6.
30. Struthers RS, Nicholls AJ, Grundy J, Chen T, Jimenez R, Samuel SC Yen, et al. Suppression of gonadotropins and estradiol in premenopausal women by oral administration of the nonpeptide gonadotropin-releasing hormone antagonist. Elagolix Clin Endocrinol Metab, February. 2009;94(2):545–51.
31. US Environmental Protection Agency, 1996.
32. Zondervan KJ, Yudkin PL, Vessey MP, Dawes MG, Barlow DH, Kennedy ST. Prevalence and incidence of chronic pelvic pain in primary care: evidence from a national general practice database. Br J Obstet Gynaecol. 1999;106:1149-55.

Index

Page numbers followed by *f* refer to figure and *t* refer to table